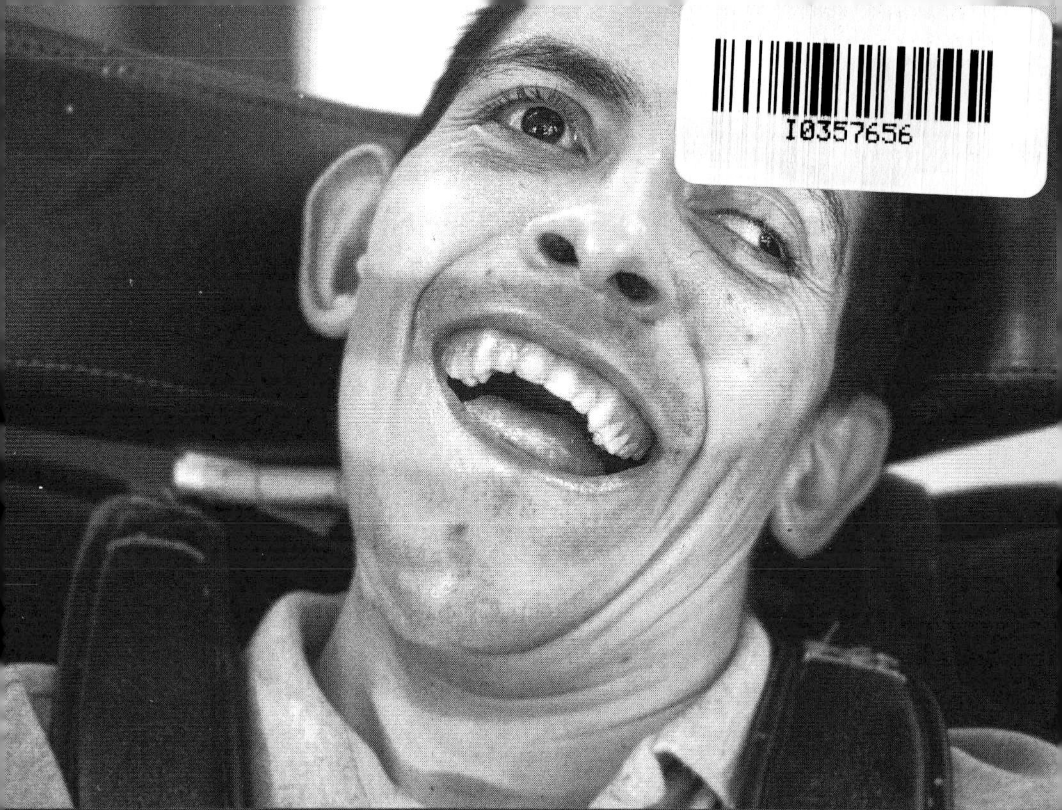

Supporting People with Profound and Multiple Learning Disabilities

Achieve together

Pavilion

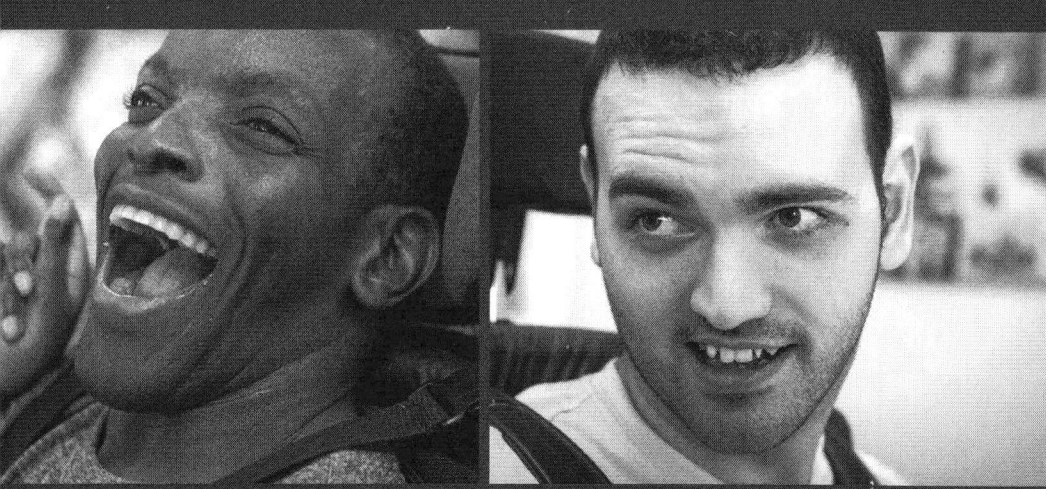

Katie Reid and Erren Wheatland

Supporting People with Profound and Multiple Learning Disabilities

© Pavilion Publishing & Media Ltd

The authors have asserted their rights in accordance with the Copyright, Designs and Patents Act (1988) to be identified as the author of this work.

Published by:
Pavilion Publishing and Media Ltd
Blue Sky Offices
Cecil Pashley Way
Shoreham by Sea
West Sussex
BN43 5FF
Tel: 01273 434 943
Fax: 01273 227 308
Email: info@pavpub.com

Published 2019

All rights reserved. No part of this publication may be reproduced, stored in a retrieval system, or transmitted in any form or by any means, electronic, mechanical, photocopying, recording or otherwise, without prior permission in writing of the publisher and the copyright owners.

A catalogue record for this book is available from the British Library.

ISBN: 978-1-912755-61-5

Pavilion Publishing and Media is a leading publisher of books, training materials and digital content in mental health, social care and allied fields. Pavilion and its imprints offer must-have knowledge and innovative learning solutions underpinned by sound research and professional values.

Authors: Katie Reid and Erren Wheatland
Production Editor: Mike Benge, Pavilion Publishing and Media Ltd.
Cover design: Tony Pitt Pavilion Publishing and Media Ltd.
Page layout and typesetting: Emma Dawe, Pavilion Publishing and Media Ltd.
Printing: CMP Digital Print Solutions

Contents

About the authors 2

Introduction 3

Chapter One: Supporting health and everyday needs 5

Chapter Two: Supporting emotional health and well-being 19

Chapter Three: Communication 31

Chapter Four: Sensory engagement and activities 45

Chapter Five: Collaboration and co-production 63

Chapter Six: Legislation, values and attitudes 71

About the authors

Erren Wheatland is a dual registered nurse (adult and children), she has a BSc in Professional Practice, and a PG Cert in the Epilepsies. She has worked within an Acute NHS Trust, a Community NHS Trust and is now a Specialist Nurse Practitioner at Achieve together. Erren's career predominately has been supporting children, young people and adults with PMLD, complex health needs and life-limiting conditions in managerial and educational roles. Erren's career was inspired by her parents who as well as raising their own children, have always fostered children with learning disabilities and complex health needs. She is passionate and committed to provide excellence in health and social care.

Katie Reid works as a Healthcare Facilitator at Achieve together. Her primary role is to advocate for people with learning disabilities, ensuring that they have equal access to health services, striving to reduce health inequalities. She works directly with individuals, working in collaboration with families, external health professionals and therapists to ensure people receive excellent health care support.

Her background has covered children's services including working in support roles and as a Registered Manager, where she provided support for children and young adults with Profound and Multiple Learning Disabilities and associated complex health needs. This is an area of her work in which she continues to be very passionate about!

Introduction

The late Professor Jim Mansell, in his review of services for adults with profound and multiple learning disabilities (Mansell, 2010), noted that:

> 'People with profound intellectual and multiple disabilities are among the most disabled individuals in our community. They have a profound intellectual disability, which means that their intelligence quotient is estimated to be under 20 and therefore they have severely limited understanding. In addition, they have multiple disabilities, which may include impairments of vision, hearing and movement as well as other problems like epilepsy and autism. Most people in this group are unable to walk unaided and many people have complex health needs requiring extensive help.'

The severity of these disabilities means that an individual will need support with most aspects of daily life, and it is important to recognise that the support needs will vary from one person to another.

> 'People with profound intellectual and multiple disabilities have great difficulty communicating; they typically have very limited understanding and express themselves through non-verbal means, or at most through using a few words or symbols. They often show limited evidence of intention.' (Mansell, 2010)

Meaningful communication is one of the most important everyday needs among individuals with PMLD because, with effective help, they are enabled to connect with others and to make sense and engage in the world around them.

> 'Some people have, in addition, problems of challenging behaviour such as self-injury.' (Mansell, 2010)

There is very limited research that looks specifically at mental health and people with PMLD, but it is increasingly acknowledged that many experience depression, anxiety and stress, which are frequently overlooked or misattributed to their learning disabilities.

Jim Mansell also acknowledges that:

> 'Despite such serious impairments, people with profound intellectual and multiple disabilities can form relationships, make choices and enjoy activities. The people who love and care for them can often understand their personality, their mood and their preferences.'

While it is acknowledged that people with PMLD have high support needs, it must never be overlooked that first and foremost they are a 'person' who has a valuable contribution to make in society. With the right support, everybody, regardless of their ability, has the potential to live a fulfilling and enriched life.

Learning objectives

This self-study guide focuses on the complex and holistic needs of people with profound and multiple learning disabilities. It will help staff to develop their knowledge of how to communicate, engage and develop appropriate strategies to provide effective, meaningful support.

People completing this guide will gain knowledge and understanding on:

- the physical health and everyday needs of people with profound and multiple learning disabilities
- how to support mental health and emotional well-being
- various communication methods and approaches
- the sensory system and its relevance to meaningful engagement
- the importance of partnership working across health and social care services
- legislative and professional movements that are enhancing service provision
- values, beliefs and attitudes and their influence they have on people's life opportunities.

This self-study guide includes key knowledge, case studies, thinking and practice activities, learning points and links to video clips to enable staff to study at their own pace as part of their continuing professional development or to support any qualifying training in the field.

Reference

Mansell J (2010) *Raising our Sights: Services for adults with profound intellectual and multiple disabilities. A report by Professor Jim Mansell*. Project report. Department of Health, London. Available at: www.mencap.org.uk/sites/default/files/2016-06/Raising_our_Sights_report.pdf (accessed September 2019).

Chapter One: Supporting health and everyday needs

We can all do something to improve the health and well-being of a person with profound and multiple learning disabilities; it is a shared responsibility.

This chapter focuses on the definition of profound and multiple learning disabilities (PMLD), the everyday support needs for a person with PMLD, and the associated complex health needs. It will also explore health facilitation and planning and how to make the most of health services/appointments, with reasonable adjustments.

What does profound and multiple learning disabilities mean?

The term 'profound and multiple learning disabilities' is a description rather than a clinical diagnosis. As well as a profound learning disability, an individual will have two or more conditions affecting their overall health and well-being such as:

- physical disabilities that significantly restrict mobility and the person's ability to carry out everyday tasks
- sensory impairments
- communication difficulties
- specific health conditions, such as epilepsy and gastro-oesophageal reflux disease.

The severity of these disabilities means that an individual will need support with everyday life skills, may have difficulties expressing themselves (which can lead them to present with behaviours that can challenge) and may have additional mental health needs.

The *Raising Our Sights* report from the late Professor Jim Mansell (2010) recognised that people with PMLD are a heterogeneous/diverse group who have a complex range of difficulties. In England there are over 16,000 people with profound and multiple learning disabilities, and this is likely to rise by 1.8% each year on average (Emerson, 2009).

Practice activity

It recognised that the term PMLD is a clinical description but perhaps we should re-frame our own understanding of the term and consider that 'profound' can also mean 'deep, intense, wise, requiring great insight or knowledge' (PAMIS, 2017).

Consider someone you support, using the acronym below, and write down some positive words to describe their personality traits.

We've started you off…

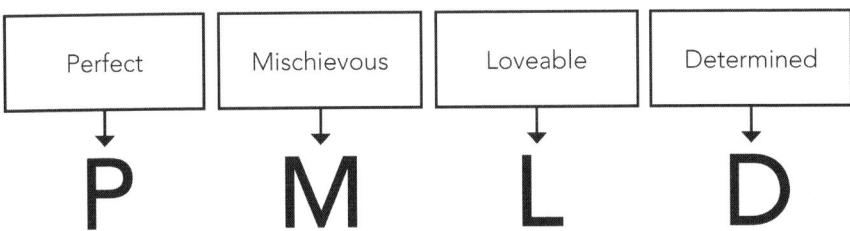

You can think of other words that don't fit the acronym and add them to list below…

- Kind
- Resilient
-
-

- Empathetic
- Fun
-
-

Everyday needs

People with PMLD require high quality support from specialist trained staff who are competent and confident to meet their everyday needs in a personalised way. Personalised care means that a person is supported when and how they choose, recognising that while routines may be important for some, others may prefer a more flexible approach.

Thinking activity

How would you feel if you hadn't slept well but you lived in a support service and a member of staff insisted that you got up as it was 'time for breakfast'? What if you couldn't verbally communicate that you wanted to rest for longer, how would you react? How could you get your voice heard? How would you feel if someone else took your choice and control away from you?

Practice activity

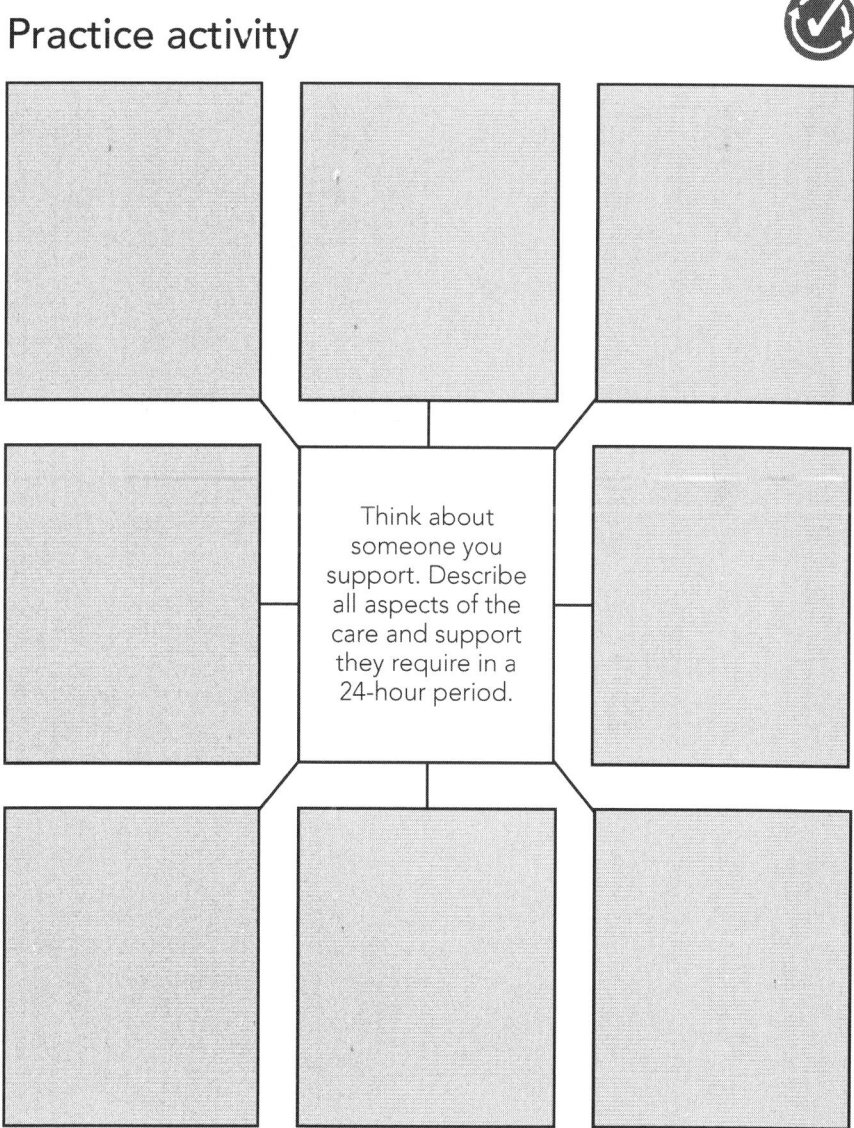

Think about someone you support. Describe all aspects of the care and support they require in a 24-hour period.

Now compare your list with the everyday needs of Alex detailed in the case study below. Are there any aspects of support that you have overlooked? Make a list of them here:

_____
_____
_____
_____
_____
_____
_____
_____
_____

Case study: Alex

Alex is 24 years of age. He is a bright, charismatic, fun loving, sociable young man with a remarkable personality. Alex has a very sensitive and perceptive quality too; if he knows you well, he can easily pick up on how you are feeling. Alex has a very close relationship with his family, and his mother visits him every week.

Alex also has profound and multiple learning disabilities, epilepsy, gastro-oesophageal reflux and dysphagia. He is prone to chest infections and experiences chronic constipation.

Alex lives in a residential home and is dependent on a team of skilled and experienced staff to meet his everyday and health needs.

Given Alex's complexities, he requires support to ensure his physical, social and emotional needs are met. A person-centred approach is fundamental when supporting Alex so he is able to exercise choice and control, and how he wishes to live his life.

Personal care

Alex is doubly incontinent and wears continence aids. Staff need to support him to change pads frequently through the day to avoid skin damage caused by moisture. Alex also requires support with all aspects of his personal care including washing, dressing, oral hygiene, nail and hair care. While supporting with intimate care, staff need to preserve his privacy and dignity at all times.

When assisting with personal care, staff need to be monitoring skin integrity, urine and bowel function. →

Mobility and postural support

Alex requires two people to support him with hoisting, transfers and positioning.

Due to his limited mobility, Alex requires support to change his position at regular intervals during the day and night to protect his body shape and prevent pressure damage. The risk of Alex lying or sitting in one position for too long will have a detrimental effect on his overall health and well-being, for example compromised skin integrity and body shape distortion leading to respiratory and/or gastrointestinal issues.

Eating and drinking

Alex requires support with eating and drinking to meet his nutritional and hydration requirements. He has difficulty with chewing and swallowing (dysphagia) and therefore mealtimes need to be environmentally calm. Alex should be supported to have a choice with what he would like to eat and drink and when, and he needs to be supported by someone who knows him well. Due to his dysphagia and reflux Alex will be at risk of malnutrition and therefore staff will need to keep a record of food and drink consumed and monitor his weight monthly. To promote a safe and effective swallow, Alex needs to be supported to eat and drink while sitting upright in his wheelchair, and he needs to be given time for his food to start to digest before moving positions following a meal.

Community participation, social inclusion and engaging in meaningful activities

Alex needs support to access the community, day services and lifelong education, employment and leisure activities. This provides opportunities to meet local people, develop friendships and connections, building and maintaining a sense of belonging. He also needs support to sustain positive, good-quality relationships with family and friends. Without this support there is a significant risk that Alex will become socially isolated and lonely, which will impact negatively on his physical and mental health and well-being.

When people are engaged in a meaningful activity, rather than doing nothing, it changes how they are seen by others and how they see themselves.

Communication

Alex communicates by gestures, facial expressions and vocalisations. Staff need to be aware of how he communicates so they are able to interpret his feelings, emotions, choices and desires. If staff are not familiar with how Alex communicates, this barrier can lead to frustration for him and puts him at risk of social isolation and loneliness.

Alex relies on staff to interpret and respond to any indicators that he may be in pain, discomfort or distress.

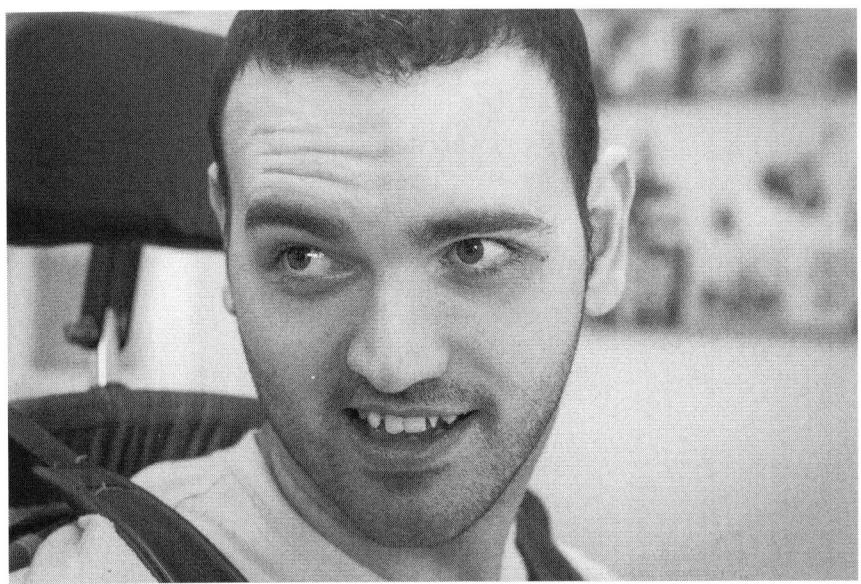

Supporting complex health needs

People with learning disabilities have poorer health than that of the general population and this is largely thought to be caused by inequalities in accessing timely, appropriate and effective health care. Reasons are multifactorial and include:

- Not being supported to attend annual health checks.
- Not being supported or being unable to access services such as cancer screening.
- It is harder for people with PMLD to communicate symptoms, which can delay diagnosis and therefore treatment/management.
- A lack of accessible transport links.
- Disjointed collaboration between health professionals and social care staff.

There are prevalent health conditions that people with PMLD are likely to experience. These include:

Epilepsy

Epilepsy is the tendency to have seizures that start in the brain; it is a chronic neurological condition. A seizure is caused by a sudden burst of excessive electrical activity in the brain, causing a temporary disruption in the normal messages passing between brain cells.

It is estimated that over 60% of people with PMLD will have epilepsy (PAMIS, 2011a).

Dysphagia

Dysphagia is a difficulty with chewing and swallowing. Dysphagia can lead to malnutrition, dehydration, reduced quality of life and risk of choking. It can also lead to food or fluid entering the airway/lungs, which is called aspiration. This can lead to chest infections/pneumonia.

Dysphagia is disproportionately prevalent among people with PMLD, affecting over 60% people (PAMIS, 2011b).

Osteoporosis

Osteoporosis is a condition that affects bone strength. People with osteoporosis have weak and fragile bones, which are therefore more likely to break/fracture. Decreased mobility or immobility can increase the risk of developing osteoporosis, as does long term anti-epileptic medication.

People with PMLD have a particularly high risk of osteoporosis.

Gastro-intestinal disorder

Gastro-oesophageal reflux disease (GORD) is caused by acid/fluid from the stomach entering the oesophagus which is very painful and can cause aspiration and even lead to oesophageal cancer. Reflux is manageable with medication and a modified diet.

It has been found that 70% of people with PMLD experience gastro-oesophageal reflux (PAMIS, 2011b).

Respiratory health

People with PMLD are very susceptible to respiratory infections. This is multifactorial, which includes aspiration secondary to dysphagia and/or reflux; asthma; profound physical disabilities leading to poor positioning and body shape distortion.

The *Learning from Deaths Review Annual Report* (NHS England) highlighted that the median age of death for a person with PMLD is 40 years old (May, 2019). The most common individual cause of death is respiratory illness.

The healthcare needs of people with PMLD are often extensive, complex and can be life-limiting. The delivery of invasive procedures, complexities with communication and dependence on others to provide effective care and support add to the challenges of meeting and maintaining health. Staff must receive support, training and supervision to ensure they are competent, skilled and experienced to provide high-quality, proficient support.

Practice activity

Having identified what the prevalent health needs are, use the table below to consider the implication of each health condition and the considerations in practice to minimise risk of harm.

Health condition	Considerations for practice
Dysphagia A person you support has a known difficulty with chewing and swallowing.	
Epilepsy A person you support experiences frequent seizure activity.	
Respiratory A person you support is experiencing recurrent chest infections, requiring antibiotics and hospital admissions.	
Osteoporosis A person you support has brittle bones due to immobility and long-term use of anti-epileptic medication.	
Gastro-intestinal disorders A person you support is experiencing reflux, which is leading to secondary problems including aspiration, chest infections and pain. They have poor dentition caused predominantly by the reflux.	
Constipation A person you support has chronic constipation and is prescribed daily laxatives.	

Considerations for practice

Some of these general considerations may apply to your practice:

- Read and consistently follow guidelines and risk management plans.
- Attend training and completing a competency assessment.
- Collaborative work with allied health professionals.
- Work with family members.
- Promote healthy lifestyle choices e.g. nutrition and hydration, sleep, exercise/movement programmes.
- Supervisions with line manager to reflect on practice.
- Know and understand organisational policy and procedures.
- Keep comprehensive records – to aid effective monitoring and measurement of progress/concerns.
- Know who and when to contact if concerned about an individual's health and/or well-being.

Thinking activity
What can you do to promote good health for people you support?

Health facilitation, assessment and health action plans

All people with a learning disability are entitled to an annual health check. This is a proactive approach that aims to identify possible health risk factors, unmet health needs, and ensuring pre-existing health conditions are well managed. This is part of a wider approach to address health inequalities. A health assessment booklet will indicate information relating to the person's health history, current health issues and the person's views about each aspect of their health and lifestyle. From the health assessment, a health action plan is developed which should clearly identify the actions needed to improve or maintain the health of the person. Each action should be outcome focused and it should be clear who is responsible. Health assessment planning tools are advised for people living in residential or supported living services.

Health action planning must be person-centred in both process and outcomes. The plan should reflect what is important to the person now and in the future, with emphasis placed on ensuring information is accessible and co-produced with them and their circle of support.

Practical tips on making the most of health services/appointments

Health appointments should be planned in advanced as much as practicable, with the person and their circle of support, to ensure they are effective and the best possible outcome can be achieved. Hints and tips to consider include the following:

- Prepare relevant information beforehand, ensuring the individual is involved.
- Contact the service/department in advance to discuss individual needs e.g. practical aspects such as hoisting facilities/compatibility of slings and any reasonable adjustments.
- Find out what to expect.
- Arrive in plenty of time.
- Allow extra time for parking.
- Know where you are going.
- Know why the person is going to the service.
- Take appointment letters with you for contact information.
- Consider the Mental Capacity Act (this is discussed in chapter 6).
- Take appropriate resources e.g. hospital passport, communication aids.
- Use guidance on supporting people to hospital.
- Be flexible and approachable.
- Be confident and ask for help when needed.
- **Communicate!**

> ### Thinking activity
>
> Re-read the case study about Alex on page 8.
>
> Alex has recently been experiencing reflux and coffee ground vomit, which has been causing him a degree of discomfort. Alongside this, his bowel function has deteriorated and he has had to have an increase of his laxative medication, but it appears that this has not been effective. In response to the change in Alex's health, the GP has re-referred him to the local gastroenterologist for potential further examinations/investigations.
>
> Alex is due to go in to the local hospital as a day case patient.
> - What information would you need to prepare for the appointment?
> - What equipment would you need to take?
> - What documentation would you need to take?
> - In view of Alex's physical disability, what considerations need to be made prior to the appointment?

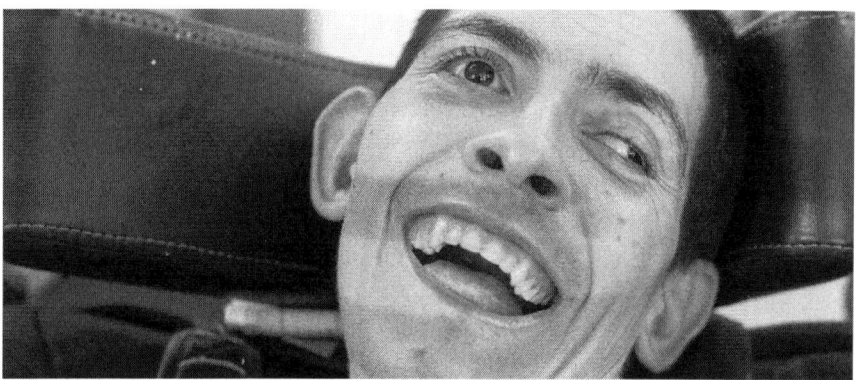

Reasonable adjustments

A reasonable adjustment is a change that has been made to a service so that people with learning disabilities can use them like anyone else. Reasonable adjustments are a legal requirement to remove barriers to ensure that people with learning disabilities are able to access health services. Reasonable adjustments will vary from person to person, but listed below are general adjustments that can be requested to reduce anxiety and promote an inclusive environment that meets the physical, social and emotional needs for a person.

- A longer appointment time.
- First or last clinic appointment of the day.
- Quieter access into the hospital/clinic/GP practice.
- Quieter place to wait.
- Information presented in an accessible format.

Case study: Rosie

Rosie had a review for her epilepsy with a neurologist. It was identified that her long term anti-epileptic medication was increasing her risk of osteoporosis, so she was referred for a bone density scan. Rosie's mother and support worker called ahead to the department to discuss the practicalities of the scan e.g. environmental, hoist facilities, length of appointment, support she would need to ensure the radiologists were able to capture clear images. Through discussion it was identified that there was no hoist facility in the scanner room and the mobile hoist wouldn't fit under the scan equipment. It was therefore agreed that Rosie would be hoisted from her chair to a trolley, and from the trolley using a slide board to transfer her onto the scanner. Her appointment time was extended due to the additional transfers and support Rosie needed.

Without this prior planning and these discussions, the appointment may have been ineffective and prohibited a good outcome for Rosie.

Practical activity

Evaluate someone you support and their health planning and fill the audit form below.

Criteria	Met yes/no	Comments/Actions
Have they had an annual check using a health assessment tool?		When was their last appointment:
Have they got a Health Action Plan in place?		
Is the format appropriate and adapted for their needs?		
Have they been involved in putting together their plan?		How was this achieved?
Are the actions outcome focused and regularly reviewed?		
Is there evidence of working with external health professionals, appropriate to support the person's health needs?		
Are all appointments clearly logged with information relating to outcomes?		

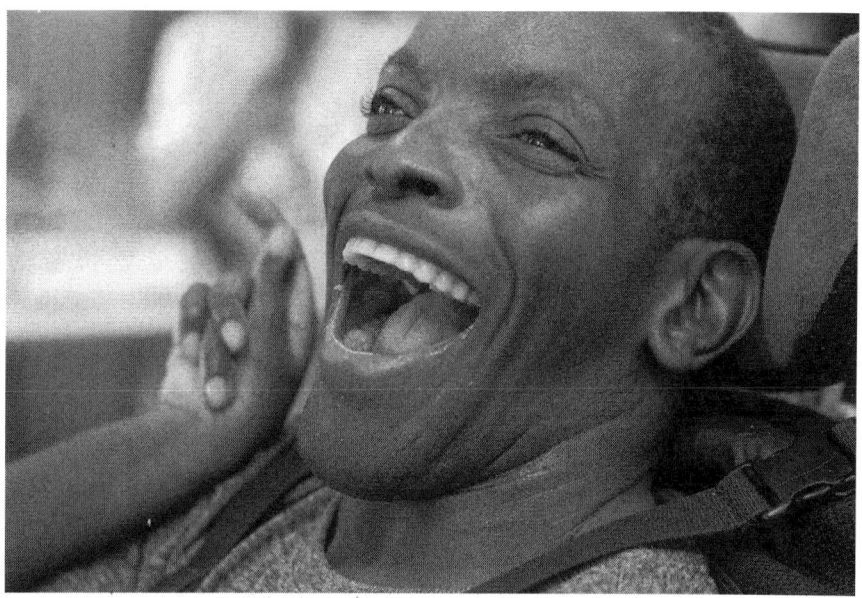

Pause for reflection

Having completed this chapter, reflect on what you have learnt and how you can embed this into your practice. Consider the everyday and health needs of someone you support: are you confident their needs are being fully met? If not, are there any barriers and if so how could these be overcome? Some examples may include speaking with your line manager, liaising with family members, discussing whether a referral to relevant health or social care professional may be beneficial etc. Make notes below to discuss with your supervisor.

References

Emerson E (2009) Estimating future numbers of adults with profound and multiple learning disabilities in England. *Tizard Learning Disability Review* **14** (4) pp49–55.

PAMIS (2011a) *Understanding and Managing Epilepsy for People with Profound and Multiple Learning Disabilities*. Dundee: Pamis

PAMIS (2011b) *Understanding and Managing Nutrition for People with Profound and Multiple Learning Disabilities*. Dundee: Pamis

PAMIS (2017) *Why People with Profound and Multiple Learning Disabilities (PMLD) and Complex Care Needs Require a Different Approach When Being Assessed for Support Services* [online]. Available at: http://pamis.org.uk/site/uploads/pamis-statement-re-self-directed-support.pdf (Accessed September 2019).

Further reading

Epilepsy: www.epilepsysociety.org.uk/ (Accessed September 2019).

Dysphagia: www.nhs.uk/conditions/swallowing-problems-dysphagia/ (Accessed September 2019).

Gastro-oesophageal Reflux Disease: www.nhsinform.scot/illnesses-and-conditions/stomach-liver-and-gastrointestinal-tract/gastro-oesophageal-reflux-disease-gord (Accessed September 2019).

Osteoporosis: www.nhs.uk/conditions/osteoporosis (Accessed September 2019).

Respiratory health for people with profound and multiple learning disabilities: www.pamis.org (Accessed September 2019).

Understanding and managing nutrition for people with profound and multiple learning disabilities: www.pamis.org (Accessed September 2019).

Learning from Deaths Review Programme. Annual Report 2016-17: www.bristol.ac.uk/sps/news/2018/leder-report.html (Accessed September 2019).

Health Action Planning and Health Facilitation for People with Learning Disabilities: Good Practice Guidance (2009): https://webarchive.nationalarchives.gov.uk/20130105064241/http://www.dh.gov.uk/en/Publicationsandstatistics/Publications/PublicationsPolicyAndGuidance/DH_096505 (Accessed September 2019).

Making Reasonable Adjustments: https://www.gov.uk/government/collections/reasonable-adjustments-for-people-with-a-learning-disability (Accessed September 2019).

Chapter Two: Supporting emotional health and well-being

This chapter will raise awareness and understanding of emotional health and well-being, including factors that may affect emotional well-being for someone with PMLD and how changes can be recognised and addressed.

What is emotional health and well-being?

The World Health Organization (WHO) defines mental health as, 'a state of well-being in which every individual realizes his or her own potential, can cope with the normal stresses of life, can work productively and fruitfully, and is able to make a contribution to her or his community' (WHO, 2014). Mental health and well-being is dynamic; it can change from moment to moment, day to day, month to month or year to year. Mental health includes emotional, psychological and social well-being.

There is no single definition of well-being but it is acknowledged that well-being is a positive concept that includes the presence of emotions that make us feel good e.g. contentment, happiness and gratification; and the absence of emotions that are difficult and at times painful, such as depression, anxiety and loneliness (CDC, 2018).

Maintaining good mental health and well-being is as important as meeting our physical health needs. In fact, the WHO (2014) states that 'there is no health without mental health'. Good emotional well-being helps us:

- improve our confidence and self-esteem
- feel and express a range of emotions
- build and maintain good relationships with others
- engage with the world around us
- live and work productively
- enjoy life
- adapt and manage in times of change and uncertainty.

(Mind, 2016)

Mental health and people with PMLD

The prevalence of mental health diagnoses among people with PMLD is under researched, however it is estimated that mental ill-health is twice as prevalent among people with a learning disability compared to the general population (McManus et al, 2009).

While there is very limited research that looks specifically at mental health and people with PMLD, it is increasingly acknowledged that many experience depression, anxiety and stress, which are frequently overlooked or misattributed to their learning disabilities.

Risk factors associated with mental ill-health for people with PMLD are multifactorial but include a higher incidence of challenging life experiences, poor physical health, unequal access to expert mental health support, and the attitudes and assumptions of people around them.

Mental health conditions may develop and present in different ways for people with learning disabilities, and this, with the addition of significant communication difficulties and sensory impairments experienced by people with PMLD, means the usual signs of mental ill-health may not be obvious. This can and does lead to difficulties in recognising and diagnosing a mental health condition.

Thinking activity
When you go through difficult times, how do you feel? What helps you through these times? Think about someone you support, how might you know if they're unhappy or sad?

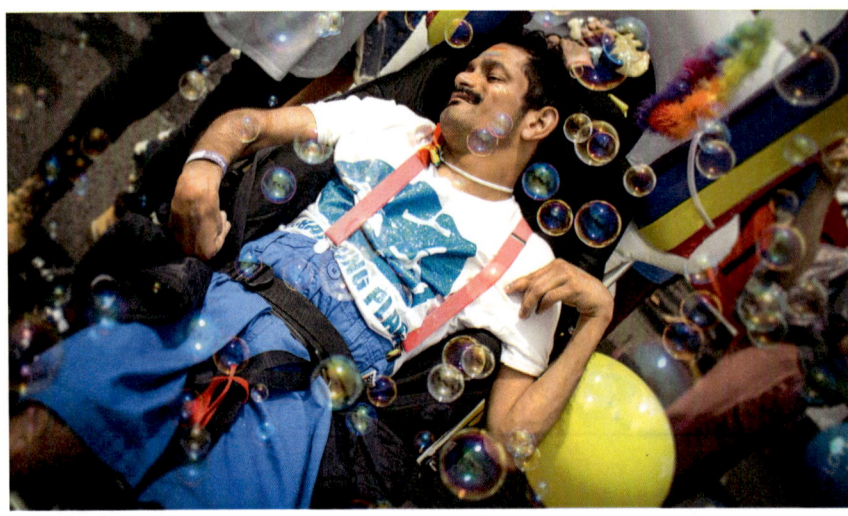

The inter-relationship between emotional and social well-being

Humanistic psychologist Abraham Maslow's 'Hierarchy of Human Needs' model influenced how we view human behaviour. His premise was that humans have a series of innate needs that are hierarchically ranked. He argued that in order to meet our full potential, a person's basic needs must be met. According to Maslow, physiological and safety needs must be met before a person can start to feel a sense belonging and develop self-esteem.

Figure 2.1: Maslow's hierarchy of needs

Self-actualisation
desire to become the most that one can be

Esteem
Respect, self-esteem, status, recognition, strength, freedom

Love and belonging
friendship, intimacy, family, sense of connection

Safety needs
personal security, employment, resources, health, property

Physiological needs
air, water, food, shelter, sleep, clothing, reproduction

With this theory in mind, building self-esteem is considered inter-dependent with supporting a person's social, cultural and spiritual well-being – often referred to as psychosocial well-being. To feel a sense of belonging, a person needs to have a strong social network of friends and family, and feel respected and valued within this network.

If you were cut off from your friends and family you would quickly feel lonely. Conversely, if you were leading an active life, having the choice to do what you want with lots of friends, you would feel valued and self-confident. You would have a good sense of identity and self-worth.

For people with PMLD it is fundamental that they are supported to feel confident and valued. They need people around them supporting them to develop their ability to communicate their own wants and needs, to make contact with others, to show affection, and to experience and show pleasure or enjoyment.

Practice activity

Reflect how you are supporting someone's holistic needs and therefore promoting their emotional well-being. Think about someone you are supporting and complete the first column below. You will be asked to complete the second column at the end of this chapter.

Hierarchy of need	Ways you currently support to meet their needs	How could you change/enhance your practice to further support these needs
Physiological needs *Basic human needs – food, water and comfort*		
Safety needs *Security, stability and safety*		
Social needs – love and belonging *Friendships, family contact, socialising*		
Esteem needs *Feeling respected, valued*		
Self-actualisation *Fulfilling potential*		

Factors that influence emotional well-being

Many events can happen in life that may disrupt our emotional health. Physical changes can also influence emotional well-being. These can lead to feelings of sadness, stress or anxiety. For example:

Loss and bereavement

Grief is a difficult feeling for any of us to deal with. It's a journey that is individual and personal, and one that often requires support from people closest to us. People with PMLD experience loss, not just through death but if they are living in supportive accommodation, they are likely to have staff and peers come into their lives and move on, for a variety of reasons. This loss can also have a negative impact on their emotional well-being. People with PMLD will need support from others who are able to understand them, are in tune with them and fully appreciate and respect the emotional fluctuations associated with the grieving process. Processing time and grieving time may be longer for a person with PMLD and specialist, meaningful support needs to be offered.

PAMIS have a Bereavement and Loss Learning Resource Pack for those supporting bereaved people with PMLD, their parents and support staff which can be found at http://pamis.org.uk/resources/bereavement-and-loss/ (accessed September 2019).

Mencap have signposts to some useful resources for dealing with bereavement for people with learning disabilities which can be found at www.mencap.org.uk/advice-and-support/dealing-bereavement (accessed September, 2019), as have BILD: www.bild.org.uk/resources/ageingwell/endoflifecare/ (accessed September, 2019).

Social isolation or loneliness

We can be surrounded by people but still feel lonely. Feelings of loneliness can be triggered by being surrounded by people but not feeling understood or not being engaged in interaction with others. People with PMLD are at risk of social isolation because they often communicate in a non-linguistic way e.g. they may use facial expressions, body language or sounds to communicate (this is covered more in chapter 3). If the world around them doesn't make sense, or people are not communicating or offering activities in a meaningful and accessible way for them, they are likely to withdraw, missing out on life.

Sheridan Forster (2008) has developed the 'Hanging Out Program', which is a simple approach for making sure people don't miss out. More information can be found at https://sheridanforster.com.au/passions/hanging-out-program-hop/ (accessed September, 2019).

Lack of meaningful engagement

A lack of the right level of engagement, interaction and sensory stimulation, as well as leading to a feeling of social isolation and loneliness as discussed above, will also impact negatively on a person's emotional health and well-being by causing feelings of low self-esteem and self-doubt about their own worth.

When people are engaged in a meaningful life with rich experiences and positive engagement, it changes how they are seen by others and how they see themselves.

Abuse

Abuse or neglect can take many forms. It may involve a single or repeated act or omission by a person or persons where there is an expectation of trust or duty of care, which causes harm. People with PMLD are more vulnerable to abuse due to their reliance on others to meet their personal care needs, their lack of ability to object to or move away from situations they are uncomfortable with, and their lack of ability to self-report/disclose. We all have a moral and ethical duty to safeguard everyone we support. Safeguarding means protecting a person's right to live in safety, free from abuse, neglect and poor practice.

Change and transition

Change and transition are difficult for most of us, but for people with PMLD, periods of change are compounded because they may not be able to express verbally how they feel, they may not have been involved in the decision making process or not been given the necessary support to understand what is being discussed/implemented. There is a risk that change and transition can be overlooked, as well as how much it can and does impact on the emotional health of someone with PMLD. Changes in staff, changes in routine, moving house and parental separation can all lead to a period of uncertainty causing anxiety and/or distress (PAMIS, 2011).

Physical ill-health and/or pain

Changes in physical health can result in changes in emotional health and well-being, but also changes in a person's emotional health and well-being can impact of their physical health.

As discussed in chapter 1, people with PMLD often experience complex and long-term health needs such as epilepsy, dysphagia and gastro-oesophageal reflux disease. Long-term health conditions can be unstable and cause acute ill-health e.g. reflux can lead to aspiration which can result in pneumonia. These changes can lead to deterioration in symptoms and changes in treatments.

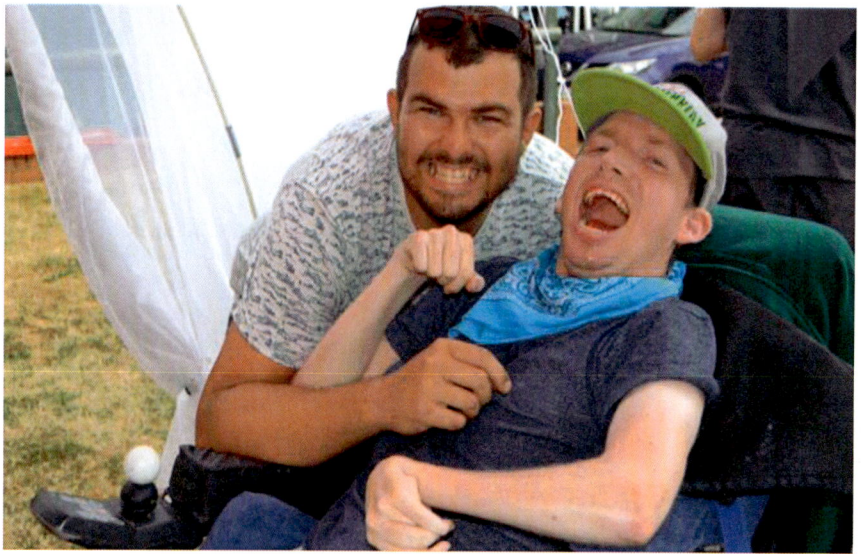

Medication can cause changes in a person's mood and emotional health. Physical and emotional health are very much interlinked, for example a condition like epilepsy can increase the risk of emotional ill-health. Emotional ill-health can lead to an increase in seizures, increased seizures can result in physical ill-health and deterioration to emotional ill-health. This cycle can continue if there is little recognition of this inter-relationship and holistic care and management is not fostered.

Living with fluctuating health and symptoms, past experiences of illness and living with pain, can all contribute to a decline in emotional health and well-being.

Despite all these obvious connections, many people with PMLD do not receive care that addresses both their physical and emotional needs. When supporting them to manage their physical health needs, there must be an emphasis also on preventing and reducing any pain and distress that has a negative impact on their general well-being (Mental Health Network, 2012).

Menstruation

Menstrual symptoms can often be a trigger for changes in mood in the days before menstruation. Mood changes can include irritability, nervousness and emotional sensitivity (NHS Choices, 2018).

Identifying and developing strategies to overcome factors that may cause changes in mood and behaviour, should underpin all assessments, decision-making and implementation of care and support.

Practice activity

Think about some life events or experiences that have caused changes in your emotional health and well-being and write them down in the table below. Then think about the associated feelings you experienced:

Life event/experiences	Associated feelings

Consider how you might have communicated these feelings if you were unable to speak. Jot down your thoughts below:

Now try and identify some potential triggers for changes in the emotional health and well-being of someone with PMLD. How might these changes affect the behaviour of someone with PMLD?

Consequences of not supporting emotional well-being

Mental health influences how we think, feel and behave. Not recognising, responding to or supporting someone's emotional health needs will impact on their quality of life. People with unmet emotional health needs experience many barriers to living a fulfilled, enjoyable life.

Low mood, low energy and apathy are significant consequences of not having one's emotional needs met. This can lead to disengagement, social isolation and loneliness. It can also result in feelings of resentment and anger. People may question or have doubts about their own value or worth as a person. Over time, if people's emotional health needs are not met, there is an increased risk of developing mental health conditions.

Recognising changes that may indicate changes in emotional well-being

As previously discussed, it can be difficult to recognise deterioration in a person's emotional well-being when they have such complex disabilities. Symptoms of low emotional well-being may be thought to be part of their complex physical health, communication difficulties or sensory impairments. This is often referred to as 'diagnostic overshadowing'.

The effects of changes in emotional health and well-being will vary from person to person, it is important to be aware of any changes in mood or behaviour and address them with the same level of response you would should someone's physical health decline.

Behavioural changes that may indicate changes in emotional health include:

- withdrawal, lack of responsiveness, fatigue
- changes in sleep pattern
- changes in facial expressions, increased crying, increase or decrease in vocalisation
- grinding teeth
- self-injurious behaviour e.g. biting hand/thumb
- changes in appetite
- increase in seizure activity.

Staff supporting people with PMLD have a responsibility to be mindful and supportive of emotional well-being. Taking steps to prepare for periods of change, spotting early warning signs, keeping a mood diary and seeking help and support from a GP or health professional can ensure emotional health and well-being is acknowledged, respected and addressed.

How to support emotional well-being

Emotional well-being is fundamental to being happy, feeling safe and fulfilling potential. There are key steps that we can all take to boost our emotional health and well-being:

Food and mood
Encouraging and supporting to eat a healthy, balanced diet and eating regular meals will increase energy levels and help regulate blood sugar levels. Staying hydrated can boost concentration levels.

Physical activity
Increasing physical activity releases feel-good hormones that can enhance people's mood. For people with profound physical disabilities, trying hydrotherapy or a passive movement programme supported by a physiotherapist may prove very beneficial, holistically.

Relaxation
Support people to do something they find relaxing, as this improves emotional well-being. For example, listening to music, being outside and enjoying nature, looking at photos, enjoying a sensory calming space, having a warm bath.

Sleep
When tired, people are more likely to feel worried. Encourage a good bedtime routine that allows time to relax and unwind to promote sleep.

Alternative and supportive therapies
Engaging with therapies such as yoga, mindfulness, massage, aromatherapy, reflexology, pet therapy etc. can help reduce feelings of low mood or anxiety, but can also help with pain or symptom management for health conditions. They can also aid relaxation and help promote sleep. This holistic approach improves physical and emotional health by recognising the connection between both.

Other ways to improve and maintain emotional health and well-being are to:

- recognise and respect people's likes and preferences
- have a positive attitude
- support people to lead a meaningful life – incorporate leisure pursuits, employment, education

- offer new opportunities and experiences and embrace positive risk taking – support someone to learn a new skill, which can provide a sense of pride and achievement
- enjoy being in their company – take time to just 'hang out'
- engage with meaningful, accessible interactions
- recognise that everyone has potential – support people to fulfill their potential
- involve people in all aspects of their lives – ensure they are central to all decisions
- encourage people to be involved with the recruitment of their support staff and the development of the service(s) they access
- encourage relationships with family and friends – offer opportunities to build new friendship as well as sustaining long term relationships
- respect and support religious, spiritual and cultural preferences
- enable people to have a sense of belonging and a belief in their own worth.

Good emotional health is important for everyone and people with PMLD should be offered accessible support and provision to ensure their emotional and health needs are met.

Practice activity

Now you have worked through the chapter, go back to the first activity and complete the second column and use the any knowledge learnt to inform your answer.

Pause for reflection

Having completed this chapter, reflect on what you have learnt and how you can embed this into your practice. Consider the emotional health needs of someone you support; are you confident their needs are being fully met? If not, are there any barriers and if so how could these be overcome?

Some examples may include speaking with your line manager, liaising with family members, discuss if a referral to relevant health or social care professional may be beneficial etc. Make notes below to discuss with your supervisor.

_____

_____

_____

_____

References

Centres for Disease Control and Prevention (2018) *Well-being Concepts* [online]. Available at: www.cdc.gov/hrqol/well-being.htm (accessed September 2019).

Forster S (2008) *Hanging Out Program: Interaction for people at risk of isolation*. Self-published: Victoria, Australia.

Mental Health Network (2012) *Investing in Emotional and Psychological Well-being for Patients with Long-term Conditions*. The NHS Confederation: London.

McManus S, Meltzer H, Brugha T, Bebbington P & Jenkins R (2009) *Adult Psychiatric Morbidity in England, 2007 – Results of a Household Survey*. The Health and Social Care Information Centre.

Mind (2016) *How to Improve Your Mental Wellbeing* [online]. Available at: www.mind.org.uk/information-support/tips-for-everyday-living/well-being/#.XP5Ou-TsbIU (accessed September 2019).

NHS Choices (2018) *PMS (Pre-menstrual Syndrome)* [online]. Available at: www.nhs.uk/conditions/pre-menstrual-syndrome/ (accessed September 2019).

PAMIS (2011) *Responding to the Mental and Emotional Needs of People with Profound and Multiple Learning Disabilities*. PAMIS: Dundee.

Public Health England (2015) *Improving the health and well-being of people with learning disabilities Guidance for social care providers and commissioners (to support implementation of the health charter)*. PHE: London.

World Health Organization (2014) *Mental Health: a state of well-being* [online]. Available at: www.who.int/features/factfiles/mental_health/en/ (accessed September 2019).

Chapter Three: Communication

This chapter aims to explore communication and methods that can be used to enable support staff to connect and effectively communicate with people with PMLD. It will highlight that, with the right approach, people can express themselves, make choices and take active roles in their lives.

What is communication?

Communication is a fundamental human right and it is at the heart of everything we do. It impacts on our relationships and how we connect and relate with others. It is the way we express thoughts and feelings, and it is how we become independent and make choices. Communication is vital for the identity, physical health and well-being of every person, as well as our social and practical needs of everyday life (Adler & Rodman, 2006).

Put simply, communication uses both expressive and receptive skills, and is a shared activity between two or more people where by an intended message is successfully:

- delivered
- received
- understood
- responded to accordingly.

> **Receptive communication** is the ability to receive and comprehend a message.
>
> **Expressive communication** is the ability to initiate communication or to respond to a message from another person.

Expressive and receptive communication skills use various modalities, including verbal communication, non-verbal communication and written communication. We can see, then, that it is more than just speech. Non–verbal communication transmits a whole wealth of information by use of touch, signs, gestures, body posture, eye contact, tone, vocalisations and facial expressions.

Thinking activity

Before exploring how people with PMLD communicate, consider the following statements and ask yourself how each one would make you feel.

How would you feel?

If you couldn't walk or move independently, you're sat in a moulded wheelchair, expected to stay in the chair all day, you are unable to move yourself, you experience pain and are unable to communicate this discomfort?

Try sitting as you are for 10 minutes without moving... no fidgeting allowed! How did this feel?

How would you feel?

If you hadn't slept well but you lived in a support service and a member of staff insisted that you got up as it was 'time for breakfast'? What if you couldn't verbally communicate that you wanted to rest for longer, how would you react to that? How could you get your voice heard? How would you feel if someone else took your choice and control away from you?

How would you feel?

If you were unable to make a drink and couldn't ask for one? What if somebody offered you tea but you hate tea so you turned your head away to indicate a dislike for tea but your response was misinterpreted as you not wanting a drink?

How would you feel?

If you had no way of keeping in touch with family and friends and you had to rely on others to help you stay in touch with people you love and care about? How would you feel if this wasn't facilitated and you were left with no means to connect and communicate with others?

How would you feel?

If you rarely went out and when you did it was to the same place every time? How would you feel if you didn't feel part of society or community life? What about your creative side, what if you couldn't explore music, theatre and art?

How would you feel?

If you attended a meeting which was about you, but you couldn't speak or make your views known? What if people around you were not only talking about you in your presence, but they were also making decisions about your life without consulting or including you?

How do people with PMLD communicate?

In chapter one you learnt that many people with PMLD have sensory and communication difficulties. This, combined with a profound learning disability, means that many people will have limited receptive and expressive communication skills. Their understanding may be limited to their immediate environment, and expression is typically interpreted through behaviour and non-verbal signs and gestures (PMLD Network). However, this doesn't mean people with PMLD can't connect, interact or indeed communicate. What it does mean is that people require personalised communication systems and support from people who can help them to understand and express themselves.

Many people with PMLD may not have reached the stage of using intentional communication and rely on others who are 'in tune' with their communication to interpret their needs, choices and reactions to events and people (Mencap). People with PMLD benefit from a 'Total Communication' approach. Total communication encompasses a system of communication methods that are meaningful to the person and which uses any and every means to communicate and/or receive a message.

Some examples of communication methods include facial expression, gestures and body language, objects of reference and communication technology. We will explore these further on in the chapter, along with other communication tools and approaches.

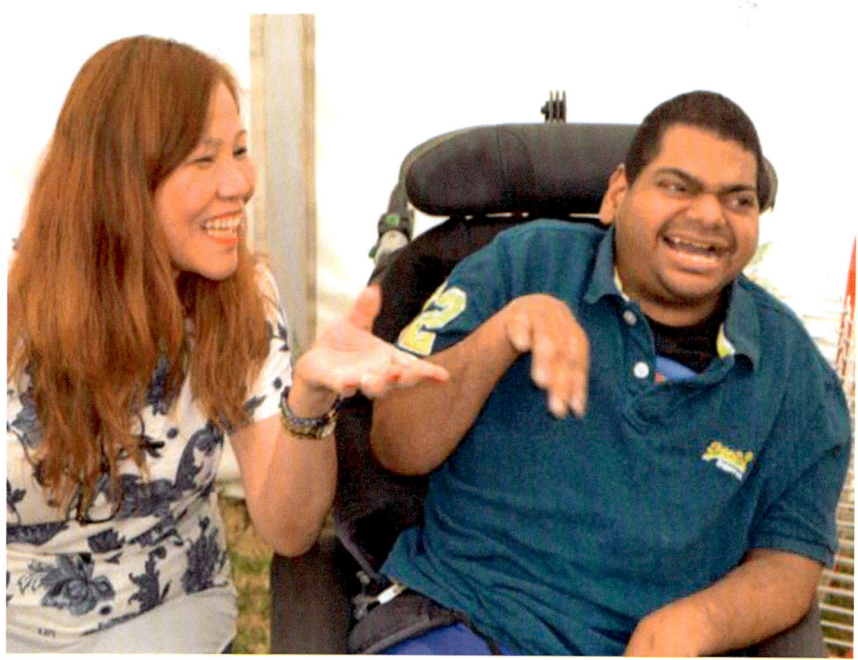

Practice activity

- Think about a person you support. How do they communicate?
- Does the person have a hearing or visual impairment?
- Use the scenarios in the table below to think about how you facilitate communication to enable the person to express themselves, be understood and to make choices.
- Consider what communication methods, tools and approaches are in use to facilitate successful communication.

Scenario	What communication methods, tools and approaches are in use to facilitate effective communication?
How do you help the person choose what clothing to wear?	
How do you help the person choose what they would like to eat/drink?	
How do you help the person be involved in their care?	
How do you help the person choose activities?	
How do you know if the person is distressed or experiencing pain?	
How do you help the person maintain contact with family & friends?	
How do you help the person be involved in meetings about them?	
How do you and others connect and engage with the person?	

Compare your answer with Nathan's case study (page 38). Are the communication methods and strategies used to facilitate effective communication similar?

Take a look at the list of communication methods below. Make a note of any strategies, tools and approaches you could try with people you support.

_____
_____
_____
_____
_____
_____
_____
_____

Communication methods, tools and approaches

This section provides an overview of common communication methods, tools and approaches that can be used to support successful communication with people with complex communication needs. It is important to note that every person is different and what works for one may not work for another, and some people may need a combination of methods to effectively communicate.

Communication passport

A communication passport is not a communication method directed at the person – it is the process of capturing and sharing information about the person and acts as an intervention for those who interact with the person. The passport presents the person positively, it reflects their character and provides a place for their views and preferences to be recorded and drawn to the attention of others. It is developed with information from the past and present, and from different settings. The passport places equal value on the views of family, support staff and professionals and anyone else who knows the person well. It describes the person's most effective means of communication and how others can best communicate with and support the person. Find out more information at: www.communicationpassports.org.uk

Intensive Interaction

Intensive Interaction is a way of 'being' with another person who may be described as 'difficult to reach' and focuses on people who do not recognise meaning in words, symbols and writing. It is an informal approach that can help people with severe and profound learning disabilities to connect and communicate in a meaningful way. Interactions are led by the person and the approach uses body language, vocalisations and another person's presence to develop communicative exchanges. Research shows that Intensive Interaction can increase fundamental communication skills such as eye contact, turn-taking, facial expression, being in the presence of others and emotional engagement. Find out more information at www.intensiveinteraction.co.uk

Objects of reference

Objects of reference are everyday items that can be used to help somebody to understand what is being discussed. They can be used to signal what is about to happen, e.g. a cup can stand for a drink, a drum could indicate a music session. Objects of reference need to be meaningful to the person and there needs to be a strong association between the activity, event or person. Repetition of use will make it easier for the user to understand the connection between the object and its meaning and it is crucial that all supporters adopt a consistent approach. If objects of reference are developed for various activities they can provide a way for a person to make choices.

Multi-sensory approaches

Many people with PMLD experience the world on a sensory level, and multi-sensory environments can help to develop a person's communication. A sensory room is a multi-sensory environment, however, so is going to the theatre, beach, cinema or museum or anywhere there is sound, colour, smell and different textures.

Art and music environments also offer rich sensory opportunities. Examples include drumming workshops, live music, pottery classes and sensory stories. Multi-sensory stories use props and narrative, providing learning opportunities, enjoyment and fun. A person can engage with a story without the need to understand language used.

One to one and group sessions can encourage people to develop social skills such as turn taking, eye contact, listening to others and other forms of communication and can go some way to form the basis of meaningful relationships (Mencap).

Sensory reference

This approach is similar to objects of reference but rather than a particular object, sensory cues such as sound, sight, smell and taste are used to make people aware of their environment, person, place or activity. Sensory cues can be made up of everyday items or made specifically for the situation. For example, perfume can be sprayed on a scarf to signal a person's mum visiting. Different coloured doorways and smells can be used to signal different rooms, areas and activities. Sensory cues need to be used every time an event or activity occurs so people learn and understand the association. Find out more information at www.totalcommunication.org.uk

Communication Technology

Assistive Technology or Alternative and Augmentative Communication (AAC) devices are generic terms that can include both lo-tech and hi-tech devices that focus on facilitating communication. A BIGmack Switch is an example of a communication aid that can help a person communicate and learn about cause and effect. For example, a message or sound can be recorded on the switch and by a push of a button people can learn that they can make things happen and be involved. For more information see: https://www.livingmadeeasy.org.uk/communication/

The use of multi-media such as video, photography and slides can be used to show how someone communicates and makes choices. Using multimedia gives the person an opportunity to share things about themselves such as what they enjoy doing, and can give others an insight into how to facilitate effective communication. This is often referred to as 'multi-media profiling' and is a person-centred way of saying 'this is me'. It can give people an opportunity to represent themselves in a meaningful way and can empower people to make decisions about their lives (Cavet & Grove, 2005).

Although this isn't an exhaustive list, you can see that 'Total Communication' encompasses various ways we can facilitate effective communication. By using a combination of the above methods we may enhance a person's receptive and expressive skills, helping them to feel understood, involved and listened too.

Case study: Nathan

Nathan is a young man living in a supported living environment. He is supported by a team of staff and enjoys spending time with family and friends. He absolutely adores his family and is a proud uncle. He loves music, parties, movies and shopping. Nathan communicates by using vocalisations, gestures, facial expressions and objects of references. He also uses a BIGmack switch and an iPad.

Nathan indicates he is happy and content by smiling, laughing and rocking in his wheelchair (slightly). He will also clap his hands and giggle. Conversely, when he is upset and distressed he will rock (a lot) in his wheelchair, wave his arms around and shout loudly. Sometimes he may bite his thumb.

Nathan is able to make choices, although not always consistently as this can be dependent on his mood, environment and who is interacting with him. However, he is always offered a choice of options and will indicate a 'yes' response by smiling and indicates a 'no' response by frowning, shouting and turning his head away. Nathan is unable to localise pain and relies on staff who know him well, who are 'in tune' with his communication, who can interpret his needs and respond accordingly.

Scenario	What communication methods, tools and approaches are in use to facilitate effective communication?
How do staff help Nathan choose what clothing to wear?	Nathan is given a choice of clothing i.e. two shirts. He will smile or turn head away to indicate preference.
How do staff help Nathen choose what he would like to eat/drink?	Nathan is shown his spoon or cup (objects of reference) and is offered a choice of drinks (hot and cold). Staff describe the beverage and show the drink while encouraging him to smell it. He will make his preference known by a smile or head turn. Staff assist Nathan to prepare his meal by using a simple switch linked to the blender.
How do staff help Nathan be involved in his care?	Nathan isn't too keen on personal care/showering. To alleviate distress and anxiety, staff use a Bluetooth waterproof speaker in the bathroom to play music as this tends to relax him. Nathan is offered a choice of two shower gels and uses smell (sensory referencing) to indicate preference.

How do staff help Nathan choose activities?	Staff offer and facilitate various activities. Nathan will reliably let staff know if he does or doesn't enjoy something by smiling or rocking (a lot) in his chair and shouting. Objects and key words are used to help Nathan make choices and/or signal activity. E.g. Drum = music session. Swimming trunks = swimming.
How do you know if Nathan is distressed or experiencing pain?	Nathan is unable to localise pain and relies on staff who know him well, who are 'in-tune' with his communication. Nathan has a 'DisDAT' in place. This tool identifies distress in people with complex communication needs and documents a person's signs, behaviors and presentation when content and distressed, providing a checklist to ascertain the causes of distress to enable remedial action. For more information on the tool, go to www.disdat.co.uk
How do staff help Nathan maintain contact with family & friends?	Staff support Nathan to use his iPad to regularly FaceTime family. Photos and video of Nathan engaging in various activities are also shared on social media with family members. Nathan has an online calendar where all family birthdays are logged and he is supported to stay in touch with immediate and extended family and sends birthday cards/messages. Nathan's parents, siblings and staff pre-record voice messages on the BigMack switch to celebrate family birthdays. The switch is activated by Nathan and a video is taken using his iPad and shared with family via email and social media accounts. (A consent agreement is in place.) Nathan visits his family home at least once a month. He isn't aware of the concept of time so staff are mindful about when to inform him, as he can get very excited and sometimes cross and upset. He is therefore informed 30 minutes before his father's arrival and at this point he is supported to pack his weekend bag.

→

How do staff help Nathan be involved in meetings about him?	Nathan attends his annual review meeting with his family, staff and social worker. The team talk through his person-centred plan, share photographs and videos of Nathan engaging in activities. Record of achievements, keyworker reports and educative reviews are talked through and discussed. All this information is stored on Nathan's iPad and he receives one to one support to lead the review.
How do staff and others connect and engage with Nathan?	Nathan is a lovely person; he's great to be around and enjoys connecting with family, staff and other people living at his home. He uses eye contact to focus on people talking and engaging with him and loves it when staff have a laugh with him. For example, when greeting Nathan he finds it funny when staff make over exaggerated strides towards him saying in an animated voice, 'Hello Stan'. He will respond with a big smile, a rock in his chair and a proper chuckle. Music, intensive interaction and sensory stories are used to enhance his learning opportunities and communication. Nathan particularly enjoys exploring the objects/props used in the stories and appears to enjoy the presence of others during these sessions. Nathan has a close bond with another person he lives with. He smiles when spending time with him and appears to enjoy his company. They have a shared love of anything sensory and musical and often participate in activities together.

Practice activity

Consider the questions below. Use your knowledge and what you have learnt so far to inform your answers.

Q1. What communication methods can be used to help somebody make a choice or signal an activity?

Q2. What approach can be used to encourage connection, being in the presence of others and developing communicative exchanges?

Q3. What tool can be used to help identify distress in people with communication difficulties?

Q4. What communication methods and tools can be used to involve somebody in meetings about them?

Q5. What communication aids or technology can be used to support people to stay in contact with family and friends?

How can you support people with PMLD to communicate effectively?

Throughout this chapter we have identified that effective communication can empower people to be involved, make choices and take active roles in their lives. It can develop a person's confidence and self-worth, leading to enriched lives and relationships with others.

As support staff, you have a responsibility to ensure people are afforded the means to communicate effectively. Being 'in tune' with another person's communication can take time but with the right approach people with PMLD can communicate.

However, *first and foremost they need*:

- Support from staff who truly value who they are. There needs to be a genuine desire to communicate and a willingness to connect, being mindful of sensory, cognitive, health or environmental factors that may affect a person's understanding or ability to communicate.
- Access to a range of communication methods and/or assistive technology, designed to aid choice making, enhance communication and interaction with others.
- Staff who are able to engage using a range of communication methods to interpret their wants and needs, taking action and responding accordingly.
- Staff to be 'present' i.e. facilitate uninterrupted time to communicate and always follow through with what they say they will do. Positive relationships are built on trust, honesty and integrity.
- Staff to avoid using metaphors and technical language – ever wondered what a certain phrase or acronym means, ever had to ask someone else, perhaps you had to look it up?
- Empathetic staff who have the ability to reflect, reason and understand how another person may be feeling. Is there is anything different you could do to communicate with the person to help them feel heard and understood?

- To be afforded time from support staff who are positive, consistent, observant and responsive; staff who seek to communicate and connect with people.
- Support from staff who use creative approaches to maximise individuals' abilities to communicate.
- Staff to communicate with the person by using their sensory channels such as touch, sight, sound, taste, smell, movement and balance, which are all vital to learning, communicating and making sense of the world.
- Access to multi-media, drama, music and story-telling and other creative mediums we can use to help people express themselves, communicate and feel involved.

Adopting the above approach can enable effective communication and can go a long way to develop trust and rapport with another person, minimising potential stress and anxiety, helping individuals to feel valued, included, heard and understood. Conversely, if this type of approach isn't used, a person may become frustrated, undervalued and not listened to. It is possible the person may stop all attempts to communicate, which may negatively affect their physical and mental health.

Remember... People communicate in many different ways and each of us has a responsibility to ensure that *all ways* of communicating are equally valued. It is imperative that we celebrate the idea that connections and conversations can happen in many ways.

Pause for reflection

Having completed this chapter, reflect on what you have learnt and how you can embed this into your practice. Consider the communication needs of someone you support:

- Are you confident their needs are being fully met?
- Are they able to make choices, connect and take active roles in their lives?
- If not, are there any barriers, and if so, how could these be overcome?

Some examples may include speaking with your line manager and liaising with family. Find out if a referral to a Speech and Language Therapist (SLT) would be of benefit. SLTs can provide assessment and advice on how to facilitate effective communication with people with learning disabilities.

Make notes below to discuss with your supervisor.

References

Adler RB & Rodman G (2006) *Understanding Human Communication*. New York: Oxford University Press.

Cavet J & Grove N (2005) *Multimedia Technology for people with Profound and Multiple Impairment: An evaluation of a Mencap pilot project using multimedia profiling*. London: Mencap.

Goldbart J & Caton S (2010) *Communication and People with the Most Complex Needs: What works and why this is essential* (July 2010). Mencap. Available at: https://e-space.mmu.ac.uk/198309/1/Mencap%20Comms_guide_dec_10.pdf (accessed September 2019).

Mehrabian A (1971) *Silent Messages: Implicit communication of emotions and attitudes*. Belmont, CA Wadsworth.

Mencap (2011) *Involve Me: Increasing the involvement of people with profound and multiple learning disabilities (PMLD) in decision-making and consultation* [online]. Available at: www.mencap.org.uk/sites/default/files/2017-05/Involve%20me%20Summary%20Booklet.pdf (accessed September 2019).

Mencap (undated) *Communicating with People with Profound and Multiple Learning Disabilities* [online]. Available at: www.jpaget.nhs.uk/media/186401/Communicating_with_people_with_PMLD__a_guide__1_.pdf (accessed September 2019).

Nind M & Hewett D (2001) *A Practical Guide to Intensive Interaction*. BILD publications.

Oxfordshire Total Communication (2019) www.oxtc.co.uk (accessed September 2019).

PMLD Network (2019) https://our.choiceforum.org/c/pmldnetwork (accessed September 2019).

Chapter Four: Sensory engagement and activities

This chapter briefly explores our sensory systems and recognises the value of sensory stimulation and activity planning. It offers practical tips and sensory activity ideas that can be tried to enable people with PMLD to engage and enjoy the world in a way that is meaningful.

What are the senses?

The 'sensory system' is part of the nervous system and consists of sensory receptors, neural pathways and parts of the brain responsible for processing sensory information. Put simply, our senses are the faculties by which the body perceives external stimuli and is how information about the world is absorbed by a person. There is debate about how many senses we have. Some neuroscientists argue that we have nine, while others up to 21. You may be familiar with the traditional five senses: sight, smell, taste, hearing and touch. However, we also have two additional senses that are perhaps lesser known, including movement and balance (vestibular) and body position (proprioception).

The table below details a brief description of the seven sensory systems and stimuli that could be used to activate the senses to connect and engage with people with PMLD. The stimuli ideas listed can be sourced cheaply and can provide people with rich sensory experiences.

The resources can be collated to create a sensory exploratory box, which is a collection of inexpensive sensory items and objects that can be used with a person to stimulate and explore various senses, including touch, smell, taste, sight and hearing. These boxes can also be created to meet the individual sensory needs of people supported with input from an occupational therapist.

Figure 4.1 shows Chester's sensory exploration box, which contains a variety of inexpensive items used to stimulate his visual, oral, auditory, tactile senses. Chester relies on staff to spend time with him to access these items, for example how they look and feel on different parts of his body, how they sound.

Table 4.1: Sensory stimuli ideas

Sensory system	Stimuli ideas for explorative sensory boxes
Sight (visual system). Eyes detect images of light and provide detail about what we see such as colour, contrast, shape, size and movement.	Reflective surfaces and objects, vibrant colours, diffraction paper, bike reflectors, holograms, torches, tinsel, silver foil, space blankets. Moving objects including UV light, balls, water bubbles and spinning objects.
Smell (olfactory system). Smell is the ability to detect a scent. The nose is lined with receptors that are stimulated by airborne molecules.	Scented lotions and hand creams, fragrances, potpourri, lime soap, incense, essential oils, flowers, lemon shower gel.
Taste (gustatory system). The sense of taste is closely linked to smell. Taste buds located on the upper surface of the tongue detect basic tastes.	Offer a variety of different basic tastes such as sour, bitter, salty, sweet and savoury. (Not everyone can access taste, confirm with supervisor.)
Hearing (auditory system). Hearing is the ability to perceive sounds through the ear.	Offer a range of sounds including vocalisations, high and low pitched noises drums, triangles, bells, microphone, guitar, piano, and listen to various types of music genres.
Touch/Tactile (somatosensory system). Tactile input is the sense of touch and includes different textures, temperatures and pressure.	Fur, feathers, silk, suede, netting, lace, chiffon scarves, ribbons, soft brushes, bubble-wrap, wool, fir cones, wood/bark, tins, beads, shells, ridged wallpaper, corrugated cardboard, foot massagers, loofah sponges. Warm/cold hand packs, water spray, bicycle pump, handheld fans, dough/slime.
Movement & Balance (vestibular system). Our vestibular sense lets us know when we are moving in an elevator or when we sit up or lie down.	Activities such as swinging, spinning, rocking can activate the vestibular system.
Awareness of body position (proprioceptive system). Our proprioceptive sense lets us know where our body is in space and in relation to other body parts and prevents us from jabbing a fork into an eye when eating!	This system is activated by push/pull activities any or any activity that involves applying weight i.e. a deep pressure massage.

Figure 4.1: Chester's sensory box

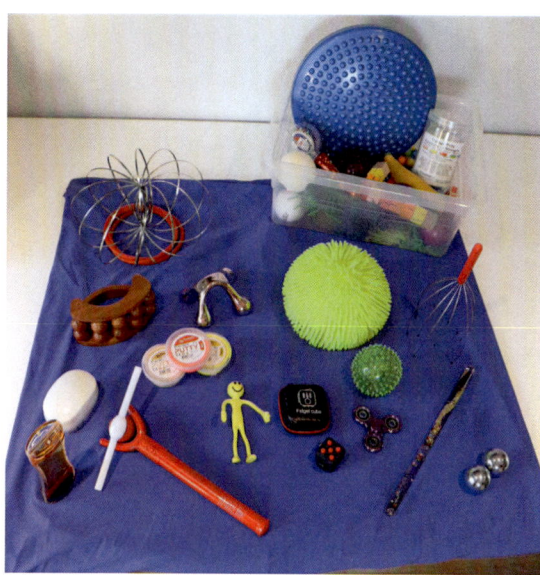

Practice activity

The season has changed, it is the arrival of spring. The air temperature begins to warm and the flowers bloom. Consider the five main senses and complete the sentences below, thinking about how you engage each sense to experience the spring:

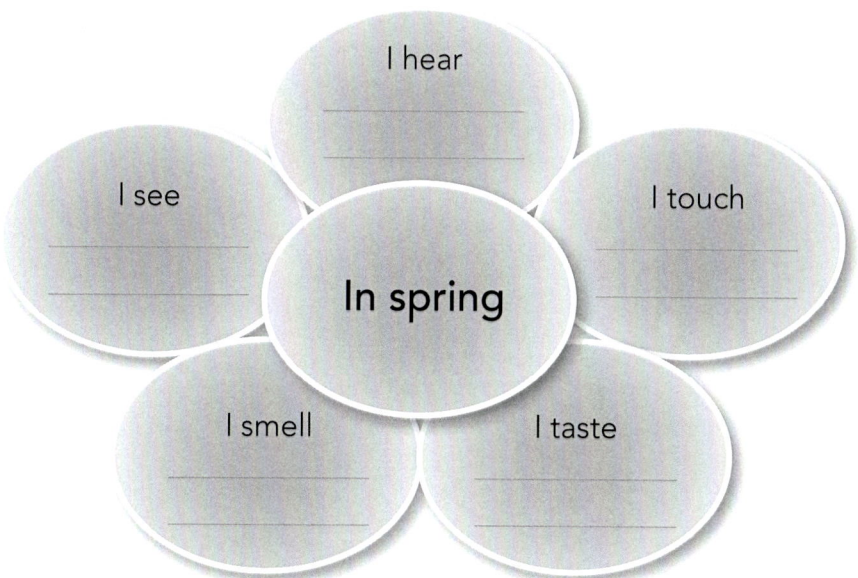

It is likely that your response to this activity will be different but not too dissimilar from another person's. Using the same activity, ask a friend or colleague how they use their senses to enjoy spring and compare your responses. Make a note of any differences here:

In spring my friend or colleague…

Sees: _____   Hears: _____

Touches: _____   Tastes: _____

Smells: _____

What is sensory stimulation and why is it important?

Sensory stimulation is fundamental for everyone and is central to cognitive development. Joanna Grace (Sensory Engagement and Inclusion Specialist) explains that in order to understand why sensory stimulation is important we first have to understand the link between it and the way that neural pathways are formed.

Grace (2017) states that, 'neural pathways can be thought of as similar to paths trodden through a forest: if used repeatedly they stay clear and well defined, but if used rarely they grow over'. This representation describes the idea that in order to develop and maintain neural pathways we must regularly engage in sensory stimulation. Furthermore, the more we access varied sensory stimuli and repeat certain experiences, the more interconnected these pathways become, along with 'our understanding of the world and our place in it' (Grace, 2017).

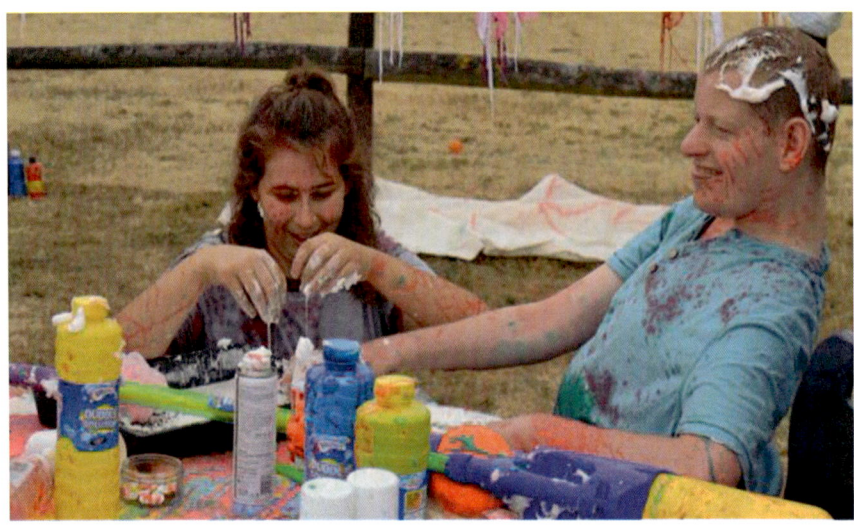

All of us engage in sensory stimulating activities, be it listening to music, swimming, cooking food or visiting beautiful gardens or museums. Sensory stimulation can help us to develop new skills and knowledge, in addition to strengthening emotional connections. It can engage people emotionally and foster a sense of connectedness with the world, leading to meaningful and memorable experiences.

People with PMLD depend on others to provide them with sensory stimulation, which they require for personal development and enjoyment of life (Grace, 2017).

How can support staff enable people with PMLD to engage in sensory stimulation?

People with PMLD experience the world primarily on a sensory level and it is well researched that a high percentage of people live with either a visual or hearing impairment, or a combination of both. This means that information and activities must be shared using a multi-sensory approach, enabling people to engage in all aspects of their lives.

Tips for supporting people with PMLD to engage in sensory stimulation

- Be aware of the person's vision and hearing status and become familiar with the person's sensory preferences. Note: taste or smell may be affected by certain medications prescribed and some people may be hypersensitive to touch.
- Once equipped with this information, teams can confidently develop effective strategies to meet an individual's learning and communication needs while offering sensory experiences and stimulation that are interesting but not overwhelming. This type of approach can enable people to engage in the world in a way that is meaningful to them.
- Most importantly, people with PMLD need staff who are committed to seeking opportunities to incorporate sensory stimulation into their day-to-day activities, including bathing/showering, housework, communicating and recreational activities.
- People with PMLD need support from staff who value their lived experience, who do not try to impose their way of accessing the world onto them. Essentially, our senses afford us rich experiences of the world and these experiences are important to each of us in different ways (Grace, 2018).

Providing a sensory environment, meaningful activities and engagement

People with PMLD have high health and support needs, therefore providing a supportive sensory environment and meaningful activities could be considered a challenge. However, when we recognise and value each person's unique communication style, their likes and dislikes and sensory needs, we can achieve meaningful engagement for all people supported. Engaging people with PMLD requires staff and support teams to be innovative and creative. Simply being kind and caring, while essential, is not sufficient to ensure that people are engaged and have meaningful opportunities each day (Fullerton, 2015).

If meaningful activities are not considered or facilitated, people with PMLD are at risk of developing mental health conditions and are at great risk of isolation. Joanna Grace makes reference to a term called 'parked'. This describes extended periods of times when people with PMLD find themselves 'parked' without meaningful stimulation or engagement. 'Being "parked" is at best boring and at worst distressing and damaging to self-esteem' (Grace, 2018). The term could also apply to people who are expected to 'fit in' and participate in activities that are not designed with their needs in mind, offering little meaning or engagement (Fergusson & Davies, 2015).

Thinking activity

Think about a person you support. Reflect on their day and consider the following statements:

- What did their day consist of? What did the person do during waking hours?
- Did they engage in multi-sensory stimulation/activities in a way that was enjoyable, accessible and meaningful to them?
- Was the person expected to participate in an activity that they couldn't truly access i.e. expected to stick tiny sequins on a birthday card? Or worse still, did they watch the staff member stick the sequins and they were left 'parked'.
- If the person was 'parked' for extended periods, did this impact their mood, alertness levels and/or well-being?

Sensory focused activities

A person's sensory needs are just as important as their physical health and learning needs. Sensory activities can stimulate a variety of senses and are recommended for people with PMLD as they are found to:

Chapter Four: Sensory engagement and activities

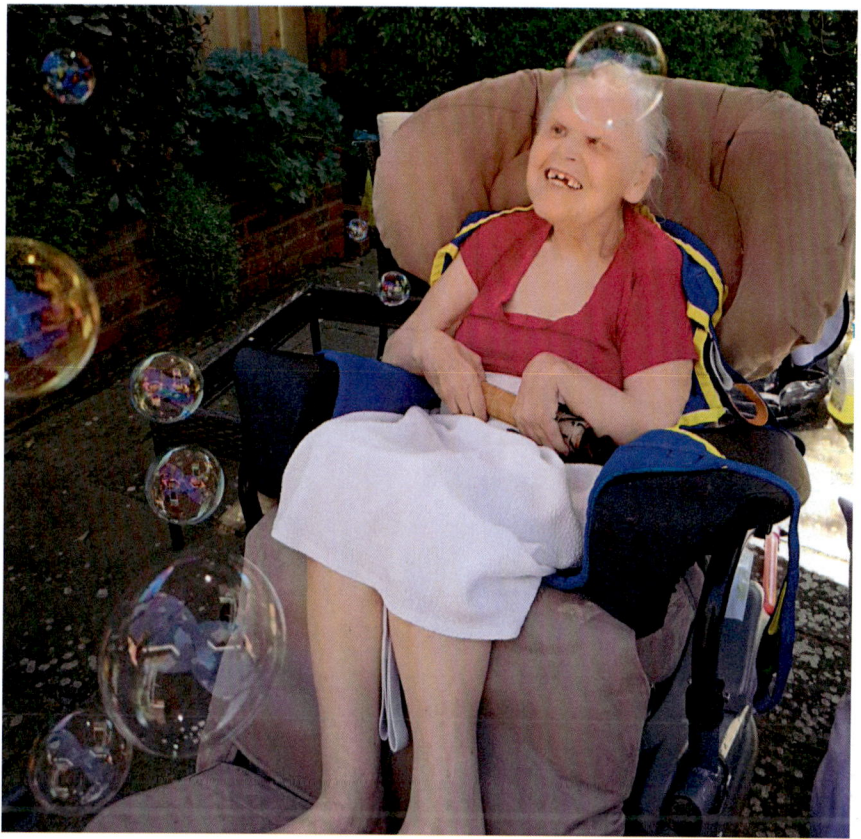

- improve relationships and rapport
- bring a sense of well-being and enjoyment
- improve attention, memory and communication skills
- enhance learning through wider experience of sensory information
- promote inclusion and engagement
- increase a person's ability to engage in the world.

(Grace, 2018)

Table 4.2: Supportive Therapies & Sensory Activity Ideas describes a brief overview of community sensory activities and activities to use at home, that may benefit people with PMLD. This is not an exhaustive list, and we must recognise that some activities may not be enjoyed by all and there may be drawbacks to some. Furthermore, all activities require careful planning with risks assessment. Considering the person's sensory preferences, allergies, equipment needs, health an safety risks, staff ratio and potential financial implications.

Table 4.2: Supportive Therapies & Sensory Activity Ideas

Aqua therapy (formally hydrotherapy)

Involves the use of heated water as an exercise or as an aid to relaxation and pain relief.

Benefits

- Can improve physical health i.e. relieving joint and muscle pain, improving muscle tone.
- Enhances well-being, social interaction, mood and self-esteem.
- Facilitates active movement and relaxation.

Sense(s): Vestibulation, Proprioception, Touch

Multi-sensory activities

Can include art, craft and creative explorative activities such as salt dough, water, paint, foam, bubbles, corn flour, crayon art, painting with ice.

These activities can be facilitated by staff at home.

Benefits

- Opportunity to explore range of art materials & art equipment.
- Paint with hands/feet/body.
- Provides a creative and rich sensory experience.
- The person takes the lead, which can aid self-expression, social interaction and communication.
- Remembering sequences and making choices.
- Sense of achievement.

Sense(s): Touch, Visual, Auditory, Proprioception

Multi-sensory cooking

Can be facilitated easily at home with staff support and is an excellent form of sensory stimulation.

Benefits

- Opportunity to try out new recipes, exploring smells, textures and taste involved in the cooking process.
- Can enhance social interaction and communication. →

- Enjoyable activity that can be adapted by using a range of utensils, equipment & switch technology, ensuring the person is actively included and able to participate.

Sense(s): Touch, Visual, Auditory, Taste, Smell

Sensory stories

Do not depend on literary understanding, instead the stories 'convey simple narratives using a mixture of text and complimentary sensory experiences' (Grace, 2017).

Staff can facilitate stories at home either 1:1 or in groups. Consistency and repetition is key so it is ok to repeat the same story again and again.

For more information see www.thesensoryprojects.co.uk/

Benefits

- Stories provide rich sensory stimulation.
- Provide fun and entertainment.
- Stories can be used to learn about a range of topics.
- The stories can be shop bought or created very cheaply, made up with items from around the home.
- Provide excellent opportunities through which to engage somebody with communication difficulties (Grace, 2017).
- Supports learning, concentration, cognition and memory. Self-expression, social interaction and communication.

Sense(s): All senses

Rebound therapy

Uses a trampoline to facilitate therapeutic exercise with people with all abilities including those with PMLD. Designated centres have access to hoists and sessions are facilitated by qualified practitioners.

For more information see https://reboundtherapy.org/

Benefits

- Provides people with a sense of liberation and freedom, as they're not restricted by limitations of their body/equipment.
- Can be a fun and pleasurable experience.
- Provides relaxation.

→

- Enhances sensory integration, communication and social interactions.
- Can improve core stability, balance, flexibility and muscle tone.
- Increases body part awareness, spatial awareness and sensory awareness.

Sense(s): Vestibulation, Proprioception, Touch

Aromatherapy

A holistic therapist uses massage to aid the absorption of essential oils through the skin and via the nasal route, conferring varied physical and psychological benefits.

Benefits

- Can use different textures, oils, lotions and massage tools.
- Promotes relaxation & healing.
- Helps the person become aware of their body, space and environment.
- Can help person to regulate and control arousal levels and increase touch tolerance.
- Can improve physical and psychological well-being.
- Increased self-esteem & confidence.

Sense(s): Proprioception, Touch, Smell

Relaxation ideas

Gentle hand massage or a foot spa can be facilitated by support staff in a calm environment that aids relaxation i.e. soft lighting & soothing music.

Vibrating/soft pillows/blankets with lavender scent can provide sense of calm and listening to relaxation music, audio books, meditation pod cast.

Benefits

- Shared experience with others.
- Builds safe and positive relationships.
- Opportunities to personalise the experience by using different lotions or oils.
- It can be incorporated into daily personal care routines.
- Provides meaningful interactions through safe touch experienced by the person.
- Relaxing.

Sense(s): Proprioception, Touch, Smell

→

Music therapy

Or simply listening to music can enhance a person's overall well-being and evoke a range of moods, from calming to uplifting, stimulating and stirring. People can enjoy music in a variety of ways such as listening to CDs, or watching DVDs, YouTube videos and live music, or by playing instruments such as the rain maker, drum, tambourine and maracas.

Benefits

- Shared experience with others, social activity, involving communication, listening and turn-taking.
- Enables people to communicate feelings through music.
- Develops relationships with others.
- Encourages exploration of various music mediums.
- Relaxing/uplifting.
- Encourages self-awareness/emotional well-being and enhances self-esteem.

Sense(s): Proprioception, Touch, Auditory, Visual

Pet therapy

Research has shown that owning a pet, or a Pets as Therapy (PAT) visit, produces many physical, social and psychological benefits.

Benefits

- Can increase communication and social interaction.
- Reduces stress and anxiety.
- Touching, stroking, patting the animals.
- Experiencing a range of sounds; dogs barking or cats purring.
- Nurturing and comforting.

Sense(s): Proprioception, Touch, Auditory, Visual

Gardening

Does not have to be a fine-weather activity as planting can also be carried out indoors. Making bottle gardens or window sill herb projects.

Benefits

- Enjoyable creative activity.
- Provides sense of achievement.

→

- Enhances social interaction, communication.
- Enjoy range of scents, plants in bloom.
- Hear bird songs.
- Taste fresh produce (fruit & veg).

Sense(s): Proprioception, Touch, Auditory, Visual

Activity ideas:

- https://sensorydispensary.blogspot.com/
- https://www.sensoryspectacle.co.uk/
- www.pmldsensoryteaching.com/category/art
- https://www.cheapdisabilityaids.co.uk/sensory-lighting-13-c.asp
- http://www.nicurriculum.org.uk/curriculum_microsite/SEN_PMLD_thematic_units/index.asp
- https://fairfields.northants.sch.uk/wp-content/uploads/flo-longhornJanOpt-1.pdf

Note: Some websites are focused on activities for children but can be adapted for adults.

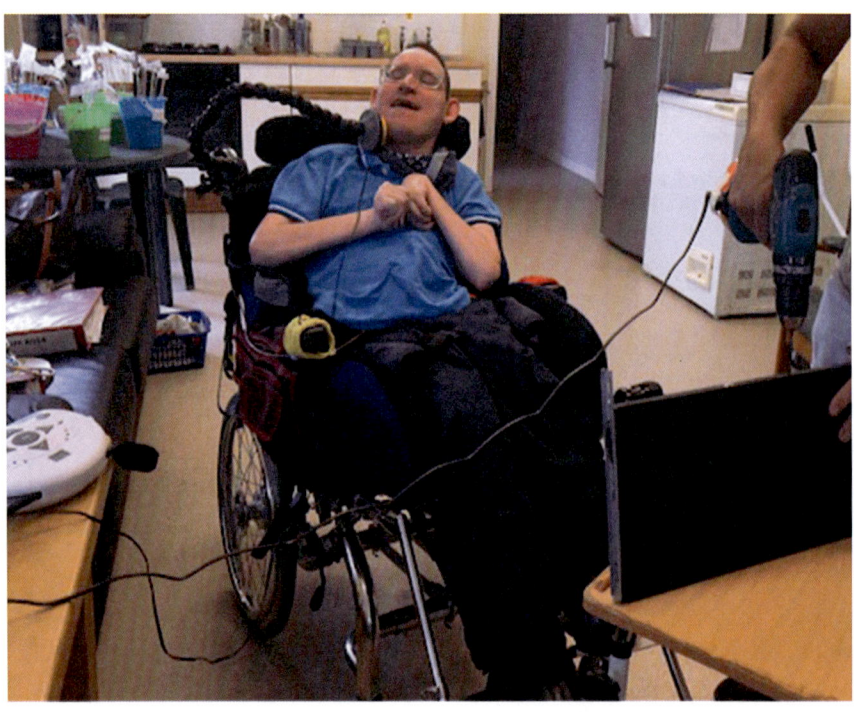

Planning and facilitating sensory activities

Practical preparation

- Be prepared. Make sure you have everything you need to facilitate a session effectively.
- Ensure a stock cupboard is full of essentials commonly used in activities: corn flour, flour, food colouring, salt, bicarbonate of soda, cream of tartar, vinegar, oil, foam, paint, flavourings, colourful shop catalogues, different types of paper, bubble mix, massage oil, empty plastic bottles, fabrics, herbs, herbal teas and balloons are a good start.
- Ensure that people are comfortable and ready to engage, and that the environment and equipment is safe and set up accordingly, with minimal distractions.
- Think about each person's needs and adapt the activity accordingly. Be mindful of any sensory impairments and what staff support will be required. Consider the person's positioning and any equipment they may require to actively participate in the activity.

Planning and facilitation

- Ensure the activity is planned and facilitated in a way that stimulates each sense. For example, is there anything to taste, smell, look at, listen to, or feel?
- However, not all senses need to be stimulated at once as some people may find it hard to respond to stimuli through a competing channel, i.e. they may not be able to explore a tactile resource if the room is very noisy or there is too many visual distractions. This is referred to as 'sensory overload' and can be over-stimulating for the person.
- Analyse the activity and break it down into steps. Ensure the focus is about experiencing the sensory aspects and maximising participation. Meaningful activity engagement is about the sensory experience process and not the end product!
- Think about how you can provide opportunities for people to make choices throughout the activity.
- When planning sensory stimulating activities, look for opportunities that will allow people to actively or co-actively participate. For example, a switch and power-link box (low tech assistive technology) can be used during a cooking activity to operate a blender.
- Plan activities that are accessible to each person. Do not choose activities that require good hand or fine motor skills, such as sticking sequins on a card or holding a fine paint brush or pen, if those taking part in the activity are unable to do this.

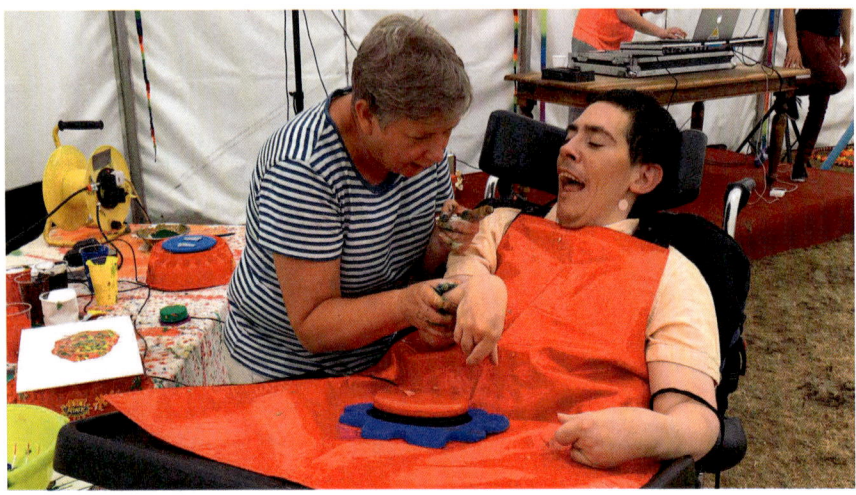

- Give the person your undivided attention, 'be present', provide non-judgemental support and be led by the person as far as possible. Open your mind to experience touch, taste, smell, sound, movement and sight, and let the creative process naturally occur.
- Afford enough time to facilitate the activity, be patient, and remember it is the person's activity not yours.
- Always look for consent. Is the person happy and engaged? Be prepared to abort the activity if indicated by the person.
- Focus your attention on the person and their sensory experience and negate any goal-driven aims. The only aim we should have is to engage and interact with the person, enjoying their company and being truly focused on their responses.
- Perseverance, repetition and consistency is key! Have fun and adopt a 'playful' approach.

Observing and recording responses

- In all cases make time for reflection.
- When facilitating activities, take time to observe a person's response and reactions, be it positive, neutral or negative. It can be helpful to keep a brief record so to build up a 'picture' of a person's likes and dislikes and development with various activities.
- The Happiness Checklist was created by Flo Longhorn and is a way of assessing the sensory preferences of the people you support and can help you monitor emotional happiness. Enabling you to plan and facilitate personalised stimulating activities based on the person likes.
Flo's Happiness Checklist can be found in her book *The Sensology Workout - Waking up the senses* obtainable at http://flopublications.com.

Practice activity

View this short video clip from Lambeth Mencaps' Carousel project: https://vimeo.com/191491864. The clip highlights various therapeutic sensory activities that engage and stimulate people with PMLD while recognising the benefits to a person's development, physical health and emotional well-being.

Now think about people you support. Consider the activity ideas listed on Table 4.2 on page 52 and those detailed in the video clip and complete the following task.

Task: Review a person's diary for the past month and make a note of typical in-house and community activities they were supported to engage in:

In-house activities	Community activities

Q1
Are you confident that the person is engaging in a variety of multi-sensory activities both in-house and in the community? Are there any possible barriers that may prevent them from accessing sensory stimulation and meaningful activities?

Q2
How accessible were the activities? Was the person actively supported by staff (facilitator) and meaningfully involved in the experience, or were they 'parked'?

Q3
Are there opportunities to facilitate more sensory rich activities with people you support? Could you incorporate any of the activities listed on Table 4.2 on page 52, or any of the therapeutic activities shown in the video clip?

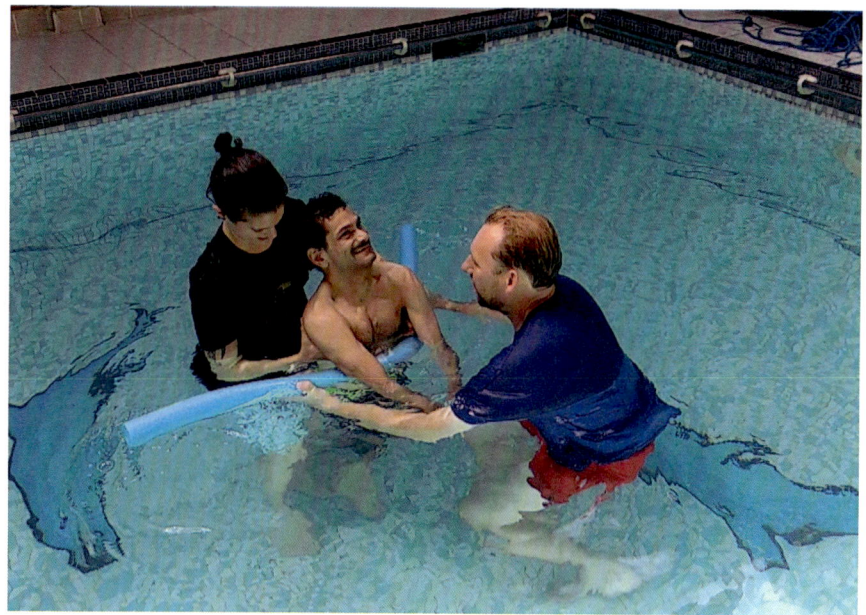

Pause for reflection

Having completed this chapter, reflect on what you have learnt and how you can embed this into your practice. Are you confident that the activities you provide are accessible and meaningful, providing rich sensory stimulation? If not, what are the potential barriers and how could these be overcome?

Some examples may include speaking with your line manager and liaising with family and health professionals. Find out if a referral to occupational therapy (OT) would be of benefit. OTs can complete 'sensory profile' assessments and provide advice on how to plan and facilitate effective sensory based activities with people with learning disabilities. Make notes below to discuss with your supervisor.

References

Fergusson A & Davis J (2015) FUTURE FOCUS Getting it right or what good looks like ~ the detail matters. *PMLD Link* **27**(3) Issue 82 33–34.

Fullerton M (2015) Supportive Therapy Day in CMG 'Keeping it real' – meaningful, creative everyday interactions. *PMLD Link* **27**(3) Issue 82 29–30.

Grace J (2017) *The Sensory Projects* [online]. Available at: www.thesensoryprojects.co.uk/guides (accessed September 2019).

Grace J (2017) *Why is sensory stimulation important* [online]. Available at: www.thesensoryprojects.co.uk/

Grace J (2018) *Sensory-Being for Sensory Beings: Creating Entrancing Sensory Experiences.* Routledge.

Longhorn F (2007) *The Sensology Workout: Waking up the senses.* Great Britain: FloLonghorn.

Mencap and PMLD Network (2011) *About Profound and Multiple Learning Disabilities* [online]. Available at: www.mencap.org.uk/sites/default/files/2016-11/PMLD%20factsheet%20about%20profound%20and%20multiple%20learning%20disabilities.pdf (accessed September 2019).

Chapter Five: Collaboration and co-production

This chapter discusses the essence of collaboration and co-production, and why multi-faceted support is fundamental to delivering high quality, effective support in adult social care.

What does collaboration mean?

Collaboration is a process of communication and decision-making where experience, knowledge and skills are shared to provide holistic, compassionate, joined-up care and support. Collaborative working improves health and well-being and better experiences for people using health and social care services (NHS England, 2014).

Many people with PMLD face disproportionate challenges in life. They often require specialist support from a range of people to ensure their physical, social and emotional needs are met. A person-centred, collaborative approach is fundamental to achieving safe, effective care and support.

Practice activity

Consider someone you support, write down everyone that is important to them:

_____

_____

_____

_____

_____

_____

_____

Now consider who supports them with the management of their health care needs. Add them around the relationship circle below.

Realtionship circle

Family

Education/day services

Home and other paid supporters

Friends and non paid relationships

The Relationship Circle, Helen Sanderson Associates

True collaboration puts the person requiring support at the centre of all discussions and decisions, ensuring that they, their family/advocate and circle of support are working together towards shared goals.

What does co-production mean?

'Co-production is not just a word, it's not just a concept, it is a meeting of minds coming together to find a shared solution. In practice, it involves people who use services being consulted, included and working together from the start to the end of any project that affects them.' (TLAP, 2011).

There is a difference between co-production and participation: participation means being consulted while co-production means being equal partners and co-creators (SCIE, 2012).

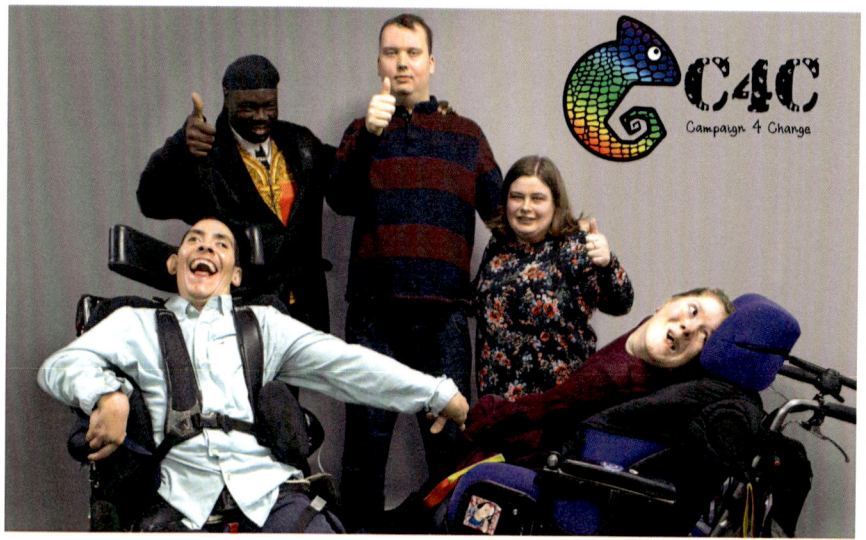

The core principles to co-production include equality and diversity, recognising that everyone is equal and brings experience, skills and qualities to provide a balanced approach. Diversity and inclusion should underpin this principle. The principle of accessibility is to ensure everyone has the same opportunity to contribute in discussions and activities in a way that it is accessible and meaningful for them, also considering environmental accessibility, flexibility and communication. Reciprocity is enabling people to work with mutual responsibilities and expectations, and offering an incentive for engaging.

There are differing stages of co-production, starting at a descriptive level where people work collaboratively to achieve pre-determined individual outcomes, but activities do not challenge the way services are delivered. The intermediary level is where there is more recognition and acknowledgement for people's contribution; everyone has input to help shape services. Finally the truly transformative stage is when people who use services are recognised as experts in their own right. The culture of the organisation embeds reciprocity and mutuality (SCIE, 2015).

In summary, co-production is about people coming together in equal partnership, and everyone's contributions being valued and respected. Culturally, co-production should be embedded into everyday practice so it is not just a commitment but a reality, giving people choice and control over their lives and enabling them to shape services of the future.

For more information see Social Care Institute for Excellence's (SCIE) *What impact can co-production have?* Available from: https://www.scie.org.uk/publications/guides/guide51/what-iscoproduction/economics-of-coproduction.asp.

Practice activity

What do you think are the benefits of collaboration and co-production? Write your thoughts here:

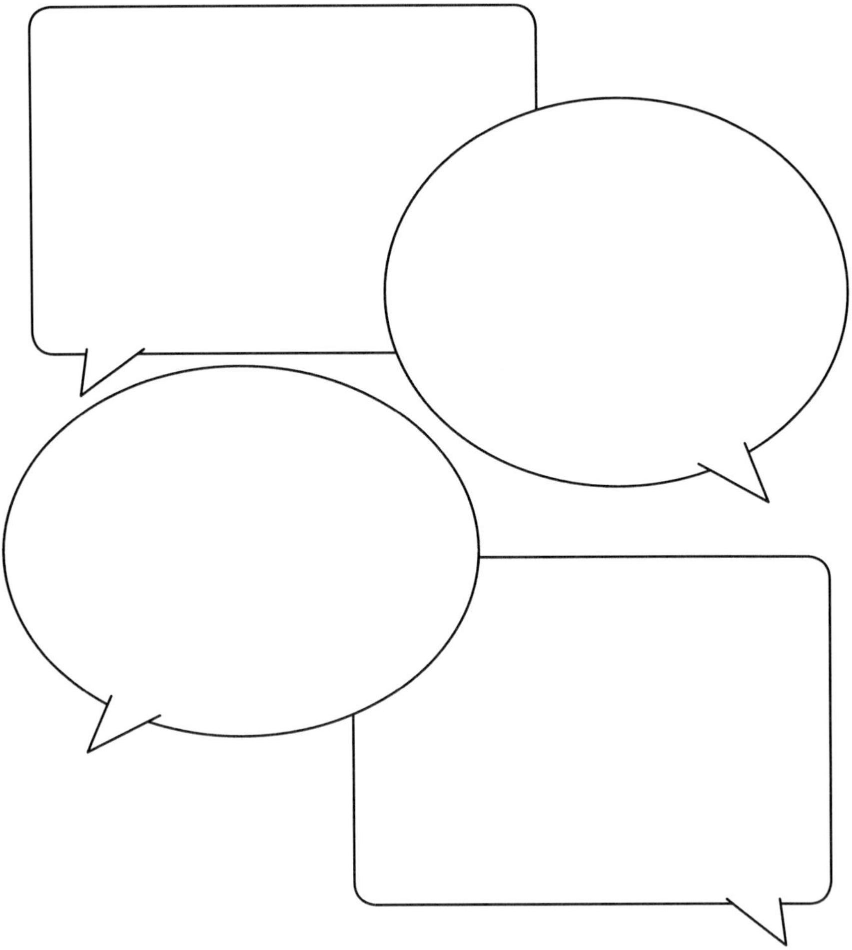

Embracing collaboration and co-production

People with PMLD often encounter inequalities with collaboration and co-production, and while it can at times prove challenging, with time, patience and the right support – that is meaningful, inclusive, creative and accessible – everybody can make a valuable contribution.

When supporting someone with PMLD it is important that you really get to know them. This will enable you to build on known preferences to enhance choice and decision-making. Being responsive to them and their micro-communication reinforces the concept of cause and effect. Learn from the person, appreciate that they are the experts in their own life and act on what you learn; this plays a fundamental role in building a real sense of worth and motivates engagement. Take your time, be creative and try out new ideas; explore different ways someone can share what is important to them. This might be using sensory stories, using meaningful objects that show what is important to the person or introducing different communication methods. Support someone to recall their memories and experiences; use props, photographs, communication aids etc. Sharing memories helps develop our identity and enables us to be able to make sense of the world around us, which can inform decisions in the future (Mencap, 2011).

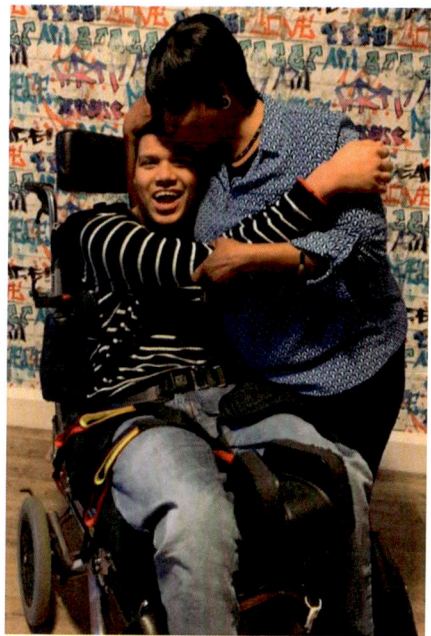

Collaboration and co-production can have a positive impact on a person's physical and emotional well-being by ensuring that support is inclusive, personalised and responsive, but also on a wider level this can include contributing to service planning, design and delivery; enabling everyone to live their life in the way that they choose.

How to foster strong, reciprocal relationships

- Prioritise good communication – consider what is being communicated and the language you use. A mutually respectful dialogue is fundamental. Effective communication between professionals, parents and social care staff is essential.
- Be inclusive – provide whatever support is needed to ensure every relevant person is able to contribute.
- Treat everyone as equal.
- Listen – put your own assumptions to one side and really listen to others.
- Respect and value everyone's contributions – everyone coming together will bring their professional and/or experiential perspective.
- See parents as experts in their children, with specific skills, knowledge and perspective.
- Learn and teach – adopt this two-way process of learning from others and sharing your knowledge and understanding.
- Recognise achievement.

Case study: Samir

Samir has lived in a residential care home for 12 years and has made many friends. He is a bright, charismatic, fun loving, sociable person with a remarkable personality. Samir has a very sensitive and perceptive quality too; if he knows you well, he can easily pick up on how you are feeling. Samir has a very close relationship with his family. His mother visits him every week, often with his sister and nephew, and he uses Skype to keep in contact with family.

Samir has PMLD and associated complex health needs. He has a scoliosis, a gastrostomy due to a severe dysphagia, gastro-oesophageal reflux disease, ulcerative colitis and obstructive airway disease requiring non-invasive ventilation overnight.

Samir had a hospital admission for what was initially a lower respiratory tract infection, which then developed into an inpatient referral for a gastroenterology review for his gastrostomy stoma site that was sore and leaking. Despite his mother and the support staff explaining to the health professionals that his stoma site has historically been intermittently problematic, and that they could liaise with the Home Enteral Feeding Nurse once home, they insisted on exploring further treatments/interventions. The prolonged hospital stay resulted in the development of a grade 4 pressure ulcer on his right hip.

Once home, Samir had to stay in bed in a left side lying position to promote healing of the pressure ulcer. He was unable to access his chair due to pain and discomfort, but also due to a risk of further pressure damage to his right hip. Recommendations and subsequent guidelines for staff were produced by Samir's physiotherapist.

The pressure ulcer caused pain and discomfort so he was prescribed regular analgesia by his GP and staff utilised a pain recognition tool to help identify the sometimes subtle signs of pain and discomfort.

Being a social butterfly restricted in his bedroom by a physical issue that was beyond his control, this had huge psychosomatic affects on Samir; he became very low in mood and withdrawn. A temporary activity plan was developed with Samir and one-to-one time was increased (in agreement with Continuing Health Care) to enable the additional support he required. He enjoyed music – the violinist, professional singer and harpist made special appearances in his room – his friends came and visited him, staff from the day service he attended facilitated sessions and he continued to enjoy watching his belly dancing DVDs!

The combination of protein supplements prescribed by the dietitian, active intervention from the community nurses and tissue viability nurse,

→

and day-to-day support provided by his mother and support staff finally proved successful, and Samir's pressure ulcer started to show signs of healing.

As Samir spent so long in bed, inside, lying with little mechanism in place to protect his body shape, he experienced postural changes. As a result, Samir's physiotherapist reviewed his posture and wheelchair alongside the local Wheelchair Services.

Almost a year after the formation of the grade 4 pressure ulcer, Samir is enjoying a fulfilling life again. He spends the majority of the day in his wheelchair (with regular position changes out of his chair). He no longer requires a pressure relieving mattress and is back in his symmetrisleep system. He enjoys being out and about and is an active member of a self-advocacy group, 'Campaign 4 Change'. He truly is a remarkable young man!

Practice activity

The above case study demonstrates effective collaborative working. What examples of effective collaborative working can you think about? What made this work so well?

_____

_____

_____

_____

_____

_____

_____

_____

_____

_____

_____

_____

_____

_____

Pause for reflection

Having completed this chapter, reflect on what you have learnt and how you can embed this into your practice.

Have there been any challenges or barriers leading to ineffective collaborative working, and if so, what lessons have been learnt to overcome these in the future?

Consider how you can involve the people you support in a truly co-productive way, giving them choice and control over their lives and enabling them to shape services of the future.

Make notes below to discuss with your supervisor.

_____

_____

_____

_____

_____

References

Alba Realpe & Professor Louise M Wallace on behalf of Coventry University Co-creating Health Evaluation Team (2010) *What is co-production?* London: The Health Foundation.

Mencap (2011) *Involve Me: A Practical Guide* [online]. Available at: www.mencap.org.uk/sites/default/files/2017-05/Involve%20me%20Summary%20Booklet.pdf (accessed September 2019).

Needham C & Carr S (2009) *SCIE Research Briefing 31: Co-production: An emerging evidence base for adult social care transformation.* London: Social Care Institute for Excellence.

New Economics Foundation (2008) *Co-production: A manifesto for growing the core economy.* London: NEF.

NHS England (2014) *Building Collaborative Teams.* London: NHS Improving Quality.

Social Care Institute for Excellence (2012) *Towards Co-production: Taking participation to the next level, SCIE Report 53.* London: SCIE.

Social Care Institute for Excellence (2015) *Co-production in Social Care: What it is and how to do it.* London: SCIE.

Think Local Act Personal (2011) *Making it Real: Marking progress towards personalised, community based support.* London: TLAP.

Victoria Mason-Angelow, on behalf of National Development Team for Inclusion (2018) *A Guide to Co-production.* Bath: NDTI.

Chapter Six: Legislation, values and attitudes

This final chapter explores legislative, professional and parental movements that are transforming and enhancing the lives of people with PMLD. Values, beliefs and attitudes are discussed, recognising their powerful influence on a person's life opportunities and quality of support.

How current legislation has influenced the lives of people with PMLD

The growth of the disability rights movement has seen in many countries around the world key pieces of legislation introduced by governments that have sought to improve the lives of people with learning disabilities.

For example, in England in 1989 the Department of Health produced a White Paper setting details of future policy. The Caring People White Paper underlined the government's commitment to developing local services for people with learning disabilities. It was this White Paper that led to the development of the NHS and Community Care Act (1990).

This act was the first legal measure introduced and was the catalyst for the closure of long stay institutions. It placed an emphasis on the development of community provision, smaller residential services, domiciliary care and day services, and increased personalisation and independence. This act has had a huge and positive impact on the lives of people with PMLD. It shaped the values in our society today; inclusion, choice, respect and quality of life.

It was the foundation for many other legislative policies and acts that have been developed to improve the lives and outcomes of people with learning disabilities.

Practice activity

Research some of the key acts and legislative policies in your own country that have had a positive impact in the lives of people with PMLD, and jot down your findings in the table below. (We have included a number of English laws and policies in the left-hand column, but you can include those that relate to the country you are working in.)

Legislation	Key principle(s)	How has it impacted on the lives of people with PMLD?
NHS and Community Care Act (1990)		
Valuing People (2001) and valuing People Now (2009)		
Equality Act (2010)		
Transforming Care: A national response from Winterbourne View (2012)		
Care Act (2014)		
NHS Long Term Plan: Learning Disability and Autism (2019)		
The Mental Capacity (amendment) Act 2019 Including Liberty Protection Safeguards		

Movements and campaigns shaping support and raising standards

Society is becoming ever more inclusive – opportunity to attend mainstream schools, accessible business premises, and involvement in the community has promoted equality, respect and inclusiveness. Government reforms have allowed for greater education and increasing awareness of the rights of people with learning disabilities and this has improved the negative attitudes and assumptions that have discriminated people with learning disabilities for so long.

However, people with PMLD are still living restrictive lives, often struggling to access public transport, accessing buildings, getting jobs etc.

The lack of suitable changing facilities in toilets in the community is one of the most restrictive problems for people with PMLD, limiting opportunities to enjoy the day-to-day activities many of us take for granted. Campaigns such as 'Changing Places' enable people with PMLD to get out and about for longer periods of time and access community activities. However, they do need greater funding and a bigger profile to get more places to offer toilets and changing facilities with enough space and the right equipment, including a height adjustable changing bench and a hoist. For more information visit www.changing-places.org/.

Stay Up Late is a charity formed in recognition that many people with learning disabilities have their evening cut short because of inflexible rotas for support staff. The Stay Up Late campaign promotes the rights of people with learning disabilities to have a full and active social life and be able to live the lifestyle they want to live. For more information visit https://stayuplate.org/the-stay-up-late-campaign/.

Mencap's 'Treat me well' campaign is working to transform how the NHS treats people with a learning disability in hospital. They have developed a number of resources to improve the experiences that people with PMLD, their support staff and the healthcare workers treating them, have in hospital. Resources are available at www.mencap.org.uk/getinvolved/campaign-mencap/focus-people-profound-and-multiple-learning-disabilities-pmld#resources.

PAMIS is a leading organisation in Scotland that promotes a more inclusive society. They are responsive to the needs of the people with PMLD in innovative and creative ways. They provide support for people with PMLD, their families and professionals working with them. For more information visit http://pamis.org.uk/.

Core and Essential Service Standards for people with PMLD

Michael Fullerton (Achieve Together), Joanna Grace (Sensory Projects), Thomas Doukas (Choice Support) and Annie Fergusson (Family Carer/PMLD Link) instigated and developed a set of service standards for the support of children and adults with PMLD in educational/health and social care settings[1]. It was evident to them that there was little political interest in this population of people and no specific consideration of their needs since the *Raising our Sights* report (Mansell, 2010).

The standards, developed in the absence of any agreed national standards, were developed following consultation with a range of stakeholders including family carers. To launch the standards, the four created a national conference, 'Raising the Bar', which is now an annual event. For further details, join the Community of Practice Facebook page at: https://en-gb.facebook.com/groups/138188023527963/.

The standards are now in use in many settings across the UK and other parts of the world, and are focused on people with PMLD enjoying a good quality of life. They focus on what should be in place within the organisation, and what should be in place for the person with PMLD to have a full, healthy and active life and be part of their community. The standards have been endorsed by NHS England and Norman Lamb, MP.

In relation to the individual, the standards set expectations on:
- Communication.
- Health and well-being.
- Meaningful/quality relationships.
- Social and community life.
- Meaningful time.
- Transitions.

Before the standards there were few opportunities to network or share good practice in relation to people with PMLD, and they have achieved a lot to inspire improved practice and enhance lives.

Over the past 50 years there have been great strides and improvements to policy, legislation and service provision, and society has a better understanding of and more positive attitudes towards people with a learning disability. However, inequalities still exist so we are not as progressive as we could be and more change is needed.

---

1 These are available at www.pmldlink.org.uk/wp-content/uploads/2017/11/Standards-PMLD-h-web.pdf (accessed September 2019).

Chapter Six: Legislation, values and attitudes

Practice activity

What societal and environmental improvements do you think are still needed to ensure that people with PMLD can live an 'ordinary life', and what contribution would you be able to pledge to make a difference. Write your thoughts here:

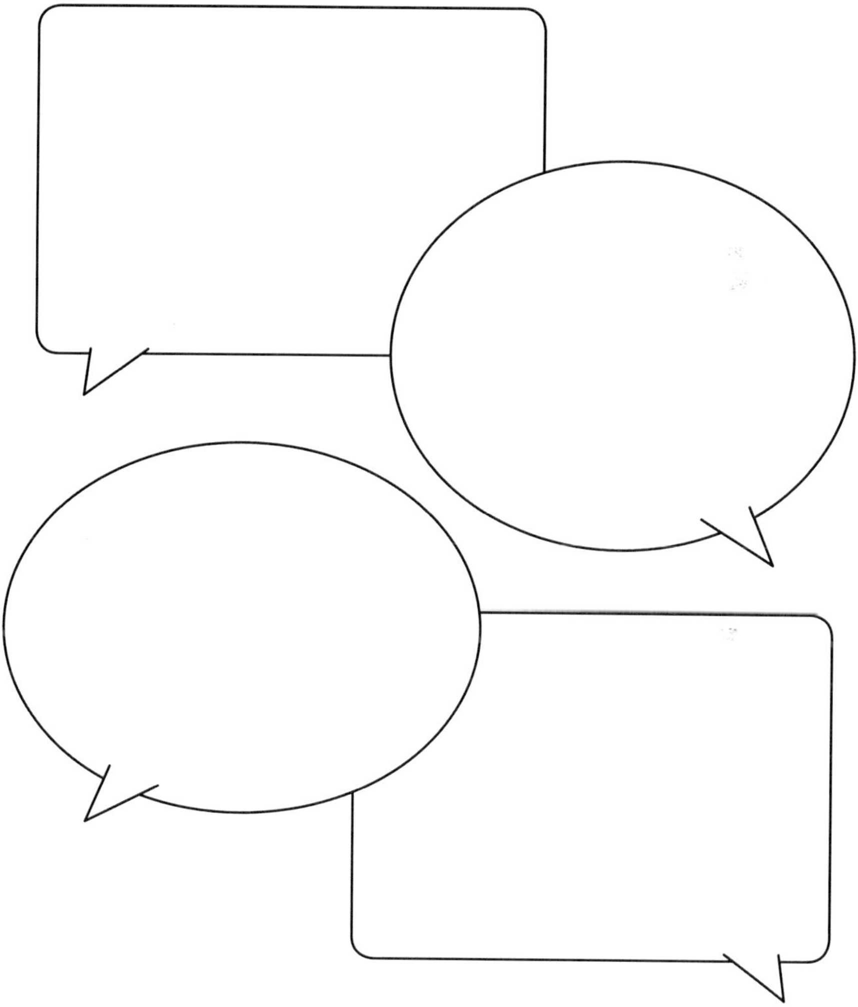

Values, beliefs and attitudes

To provide effective holistic care and support for people with PMLD it is paramount that support staff have the right values, beliefs and attitudes. Within this section we start to think about values, beliefs and attitudes and how these can positively or negatively impact upon yours and others' views about people with PMLD, including the quality of support provided.

Definitions from the Oxford English Dictionary:

- A value is 'something we judge to be important in life'.
- A belief is 'something we believe to be true'.
- Attitudes are 'feelings and opinions we have about something', demonstrated by our behaviour (what we say and do) and based on our beliefs and values.

For example:

- Equality is important **(Value)**.
- Everybody, regardless of disability, must be given equal opportunities to lead fulfilling lives **(Belief)**.
- It is disappointing when people with PMLD are not afforded equal opportunities to lead healthy fulfilling lives. We work collaboratively with colleagues to seek ways to change this. **(Attitude & Behaviour)**.

Does what you believe influence how you support people?

Research has shown that a powerful factor influencing the quality of direct support a person with a learning disability receives is the attitude of support workers (Mansell *et al*, 2008). Furthermore, attitudes can also affect the way support workers engage with families, colleagues and members of the public. Throughout this study guide we recognise that people with PMLD are unique individuals, and likewise so are you! We are all diverse people with different experiences, values, beliefs and attitudes. Our background, culture, education, upbringing and relationships all play a part in the way we perceive the world around us.

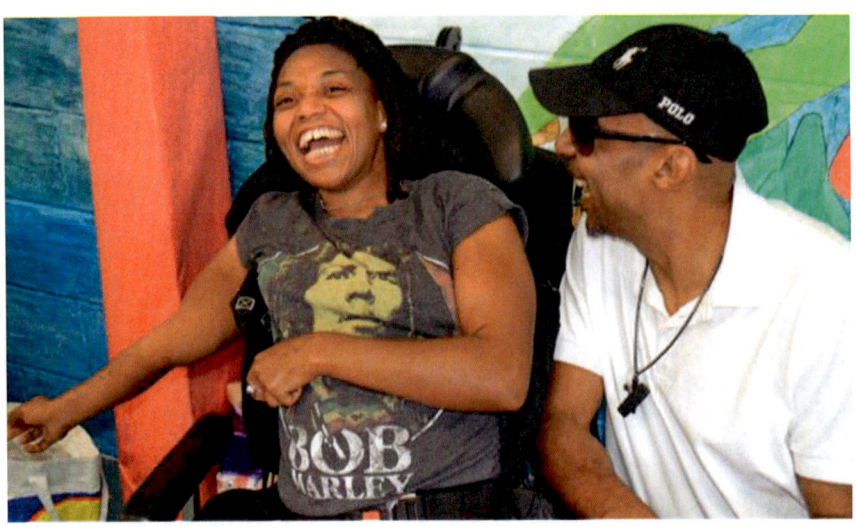

Chapter Six: Legislation, values and attitudes

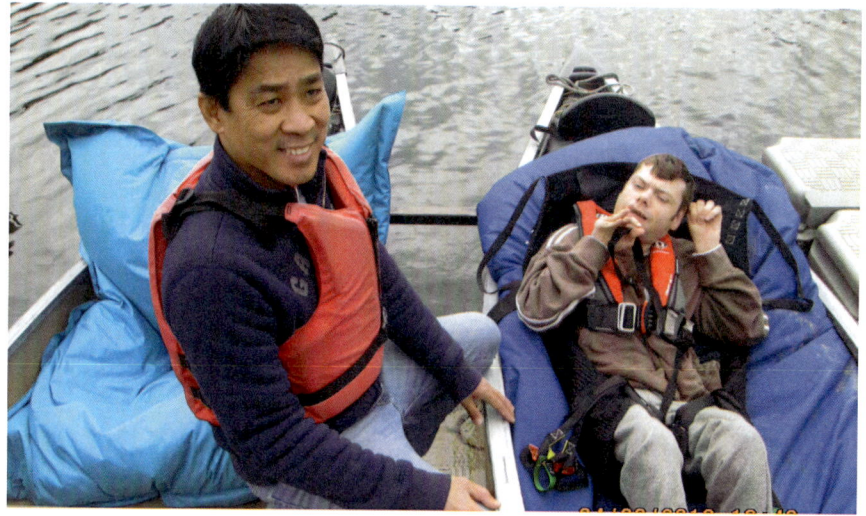

However, you need to be mindful when applying your values and beliefs to your work, as sometimes attitudes could lead us to assume things about people we support that are not right. You need to be self-aware to ensure this doesn't happen (Skills for Care). As a support worker you need to take time to learn and understand the different values, beliefs and attitudes of others, so you can work with individuals and their families that takes these into account (Skills for Care). Furthermore, as a support worker you are in a powerful position to promote the strengths of people you support. You can be part of the movement that aims to continue to challenge negative assumptions about people with learning disabilities shifting attitudes from negative to positive.

Values that support people with PMLD
- Be recognised as a person first.
- Have choices, control and be involved in decisions in their life.
- Enjoy a fulfilling healthy life.
- Be part of a community.
- Be supported to make new friends.
- Have opportunities to experience and achieve new things.
- Be as independent as possible.
- Enjoy relationships with friends and family.
- Be respected and treated as an individual.

Practice activity

As individuals we recognise that we all have different beliefs and values based on our experiences. However, there are lots of values, attitudes and behaviours that social care workers need in order to provide high-quality care.

Think about the terms 'values', 'attitudes' and 'behaviours' and how they apply to your role. Identify three values that you need as a social care worker and think about how they are relevant to your role. We have given an example to start you off.

Value	How does this value inform your practice ?
Empathy	This value is important because it helps us understand how others are feeling so we can respond appropriately. Empathy is more meaningful and powerful than sympathy. With empathy, people feel valued and respected; promoting engagement and empowerment.
1.	
2.	
3.	

How might a person's values affect the way we behave?

Chapter Six: Legislation, values and attitudes

How could attitudes and behaviour affect quality of care and support?

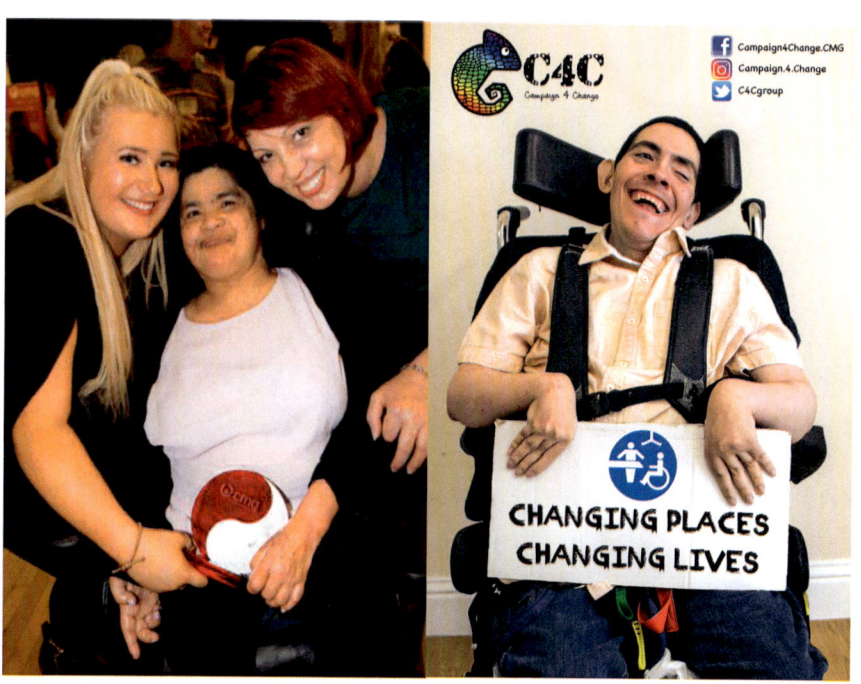

Adult social care 'Code of Conduct'

In the health and social care sector there is a 'Code of Conduct for Healthcare Support Workers and Adult Social Care Workers in England'. This outlines the moral and ethical standards expected for all health and social care workers. The following code promotes best practice and aims to ensure staff provide high-quality compassionate heath care, care and support.

1. Be **accountable** by making sure you can answer for your actions or **omissions**.
2. **Promote** and **uphold** the privacy, **dignity**, **rights**, health and **well-being** of people who use health and care services and their carers at all times.
3. Work in **collaboration** with your colleagues to ensure the delivery of high quality, safe and compassionate healthcare, care and support.
4. Communicate in an open and **effective** way to promote the health, safety and well-being of people who use health and care services and their carers.
5. Respect a person's right to confidentiality.
6. Strive to improve the quality of healthcare, care and support through **continuing professional development**.
7. Uphold and promote equality, **diversity** and inclusion.

In Wales there is a similar Code of Practice and Guidance. Essentially both codes put the well-being of the individual at the centre of decisions about their care and support. For more information, see www.Socialcare.Wales

How can you provide effective support to reduce negative attitudes?

- If you practice within the above Codes of Conducts you can be confident you are supporting people with learning disabilities/PMLD effectively.
- The emphasis must always be about the person so they remain at the 'centre' of their life, ensuring their health, social and emotional needs are fulfilled in a way that is meaningful to each individual.
- Challenge others who promote people with PMLD in a negative light, flip the narrative and focus on what people can do!
- Be genuine and promote people's strengths, be proud of people's achievements however big or small.
- Think about how you may introduce the person to another and the language you use.
- When describing a person to colleagues, don't list their medical condition(s) first, describe the person's qualities, strengths and personality; remember the person is just that, a person first… diagnosis second!

- Use legislation to the person's advantage to break down barriers and challenge negative assumptions.

> ### Thinking activity
> Read the scenarios below and then think about the questions that follow
> 1. In his Health Action Plan, Jalil is described as 'Blind, peg fed and epileptic'.
> 2. Josie came home from college and staff read her day book with her. The entry noted she had enjoyed taking part in yoga. Her support worker laughs with a colleague and in Josie's presence said, 'Yoga, how can she do that in a wheelchair?'
> 3. 'I've done Joe.' This was expressed by a support worker to indicate he had supported Joe with his personal care.
> 4. At the dinner table a staff member handed over that Clara was on her third day without a bowel movement and she needed a suppository.
> 5. A member of staff is supporting Rachel with shopping. The shop assistant approach Rachel with a smile and said, 'Oh your poor soul. What's wrong with her?'
>
> - Do these scenarios present the person in a positive or negative way?
> - What do you think and feel about each scenario?
> - How do you think the attitudes of others impact on the person and quality of support?

To conclude this chapter, re-visit the PMLD acronym activity you completed in chapter one on page 6, where we used the acronym to encourage you to describe the personality of a person you support. Now use the acronym to describe what you learn, achieve and gain from people you support and what they can teach us about ourselves?

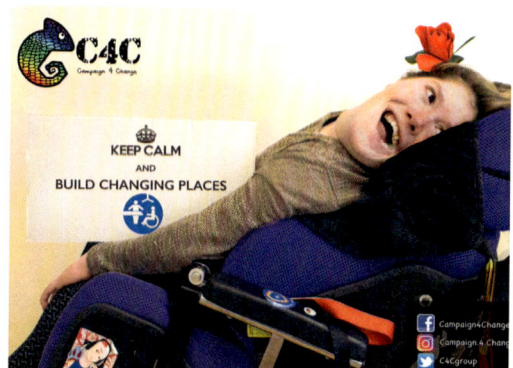

We have started you off.

Chapter Six: Legislation, values and attitudes

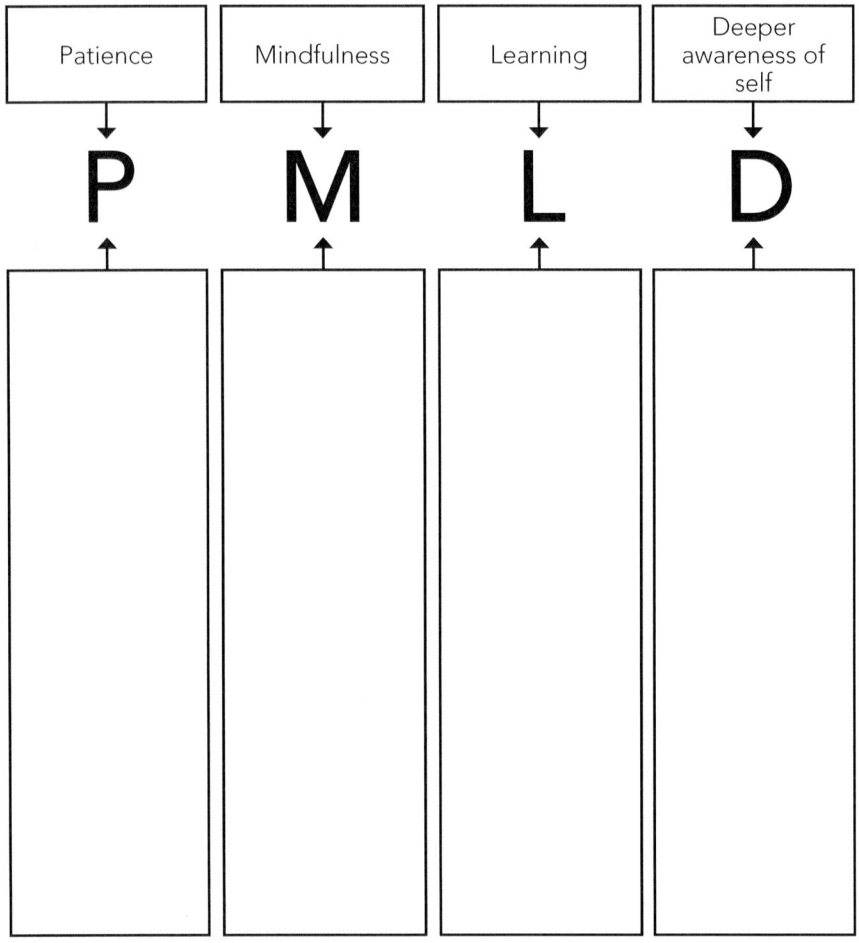

You can think of other words that don't fit the acronym to describe what you learn and gain from the people you support – add them to list below...

- Kindness
- Interpreting body language
- Appreciation
- _____
- _____
- _____

- Warmth towards others
- Acceptance of self
- _____
- _____
- _____

Pause for reflection

Having completed this chapter, reflect on what you have learnt, and how you can embed this into your practice.

Are there any challenges or barriers restricting the life of anyone you are supporting, and if so, what can you do to try and overcome these?

Make notes below to discuss with your supervisor.

References

Changing Places (2019) *Toilet Map* [online]. Available at: http://changingplaces.uktoiletmap.org/ (accessed September 2019).

Doukas T, Fergusson A, Fullerton M & Grace J (2017) *Supporting people with profound and multiple learning disabilities: Core & Essential Service Standards (1st ed)*. Available at: www.pmldlink.org.uk/wp-content/uploads/2017/11/Standards-PMLD-h-web.pdf (accessed September 2019).

HM Government Legislation. Available at: www.legislation.gov.uk/

Mansell J, Beadle-Brown J, Whelton R, Beckett C & Hutchinson A (2008) *Effect of Service Structure and Organisation on Staff Care Practices in Small Community Homes for People with Intellectual Disabilities*.

Mansell J (2010) *Raising our sights: services for adults with profound intellectual and multiple disabilities*. London: Department of Health.

Mencap (2019) *Profound and Multiple Learning Disabilities* [online]. Available at: www.mencap.org.uk/advice-and-support/profound-and-multiple-learning-disabilities-pmld (accessed September 2019).

NHS (2019) *Long Term Plan: Learning disability and autism*. Available at: www.longtermplan.nhs.uk/areas-of-work/learning-disability-autism/ (accessed September 2019).

Skills for Care: Care Certificate Workbook. Available at: www.skillsforcare.org.uk/Learning-development/inducting-staff/care-certificate/Care-Certificate-workbook.aspx

Spencer-Lane T (2019) *How the Law on Authorising Deprivation of Liberty will Change*. Available at: www.communitycare.co.uk/2019/04/26/law-authorising-deprivation-liberty-will-change/ (accessed September 2019).

The Code of Conduct for Healthcare Support Workers and Adult Social Care Workers in England. Available at: www.skillsforcare.org.uk/code-of-conduct (accessed September 2019).

Dedication

This study guide is dedicated to Sammy Boyle,
a wonderful person known as 'Mr B'.

We were privileged to be able to support him for many, many years, and he was a truly remarkable person, and a lot of what we learnt professionally in terms of supporting people with PMLD and complex health needs was from him!

Personally, he gave us so much joy and was a great person to spend some time with. We have many fond memories and he will forever be cherished.

Mr Sammy Boyle
Sunrise, 28th July 1985 – Sunset, 29th April 2017

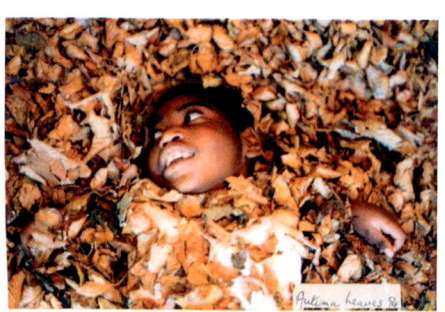

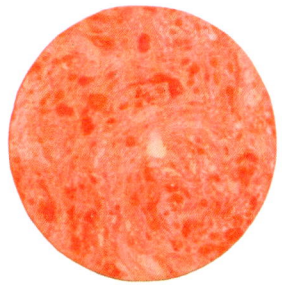